HEALING YOUR PAST LIVES

Sounds True, Inc., Boulder CO 80306

Published 2004
Printed in Korea

ISBN 1-59179-183-9

Library of Congress Control Number: 2006925475

Audio learning programs by Roger Woolger from Sounds True:
Eternal Return
Jungian Past-Life Therapy

Roger Woolger, Ph.D.

HEALING YOUR
PAST LIVES

Exploring the Many Lives of the Soul

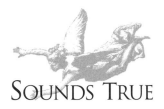

SOUNDS TRUE

TABLE OF CONTENTS

Introduction

IF WE REALLY WANT to know who we are, we must first know who we were. In this integrated book-and-CD learning experience, I want to invite you to explore a specific, highly effective path to self-knowledge and the freedom it brings. This path, which I call Deep Memory Process™, is a practice I've developed over the past twenty years by blending past-life regression therapy with the active imagination techniques of Jungian psychotherapy, but it has its roots in a much more ancient tradition of remembering "who we were" and understanding "what we have become." It offers a set of tools for delving into the deep recesses of your unconscious mind—what we call the *soul*—to discover where memories of past existence are stored and bring them to light. The exercises and practices you will work through here are surprisingly simple and easy to learn, but they can open you to a profound new self-awareness, help you heal old wounds, and show you your precise place in the scheme of the universe. They can open to you, in short, the transcendent reality of the soul.

WHAT ARE PAST LIVES?

If you imagine your psyche as a computer, you can think of past lives as old, corrupted programs that interfere with its running. Like unwanted files you cannot delete, they run over and over in the deepest recesses of your psyche, depleting its resources and making it operate ever more slowly, even to the point of shutdown. The simple meditation practices you'll learn in this book and CD work like disk scans to find and repair those malfunctioning past-life "programs" so you can restore your psychic computer to top performance.

The computer of the psyche is a complex system, with many programs running both close to the surface, at a level we're aware of, and deeper, at a level that's invisible to us (much like an operating system such as MS-DOS, which depends on masses of files and code we never see until we hit the wrong key by mistake). We might call the superficial level the *personality program* and the deeper level the *soul program*. When problems arise in our day-to-day functioning, they may be the result of mistakes we make in our own running of the program at the personality level—user error, if you will—and such problems are easy to fix. When, for example, we are overanxious about being late or blame ourselves excessively for not being tidy enough, we can usually adjust our behaviors by imposing new habits. But problems at the soul level—such as depression, compulsive cleanliness, or irrational phobias about fire, high places, being robbed, and so on—where patterns from past lives lie embedded deep in our psychic history, can cause the equivalent of a computer's "fatal error": severe physical and emotional problems in our present lives and serious karmic consequences for the evolution of the soul.

I confess that I came late in life to computers and, like many of my generation, lack the facility that my children have with them. I hope you'll forgive the traditionalist in me, who is more at home with terms like "soul" and "unconscious" than with computerese—and, as we go on, I hope you will feel free to translate my terms into your own preferred lingo. Whether we talk of genetic coding or cellular memory, of the psyche's operating system or the soul's deep history, the essential point is the same: we are all ruled by forces and powers far larger than we know, and greatest of these is what we may simply call "the past," a vast psychic pool of prior conditioning that we all share, created by human experience, error, and misdemeanor over millennia. As the philosopher George Santayana succinctly put it, "Those who cannot remember the past are condemned to repeat it"—but when we learn to remember, using tools like those you are about to discover, we begin to free ourselves from the power of the past.

A SKEPTIC'S JOURNEY

Working with past lives is for me just one step on a greater personal journey. I have been led to study different religions throughout my life: Hinduism and Vedanta drew me in my teens, and later I began to practice a form of Buddhist meditation. My focus in graduate school at London University was religious mysticism. For my professional training, I went to the C.G. Jung Institute in Zurich to immerse myself in Carl Jung's psychology of archetypal symbolism and the collective unconscious; later I studied directly with shamans and spiritual healers in South America. From them I learned how many of our blocked feelings and deeper issues can be released by rebalancing the subtle bodies, and that we have many spiritual resources available to us from the "higher worlds" of the ancestors and other spirit beings. Brazil, in particular, has a very advanced spiritual psychology of past lives derived from the widespread spiritualist practice called Kardecism. In recent years, I have continued to work in Brazil, training therapists in Deep Memory Process, and I remain quite close to that country's Umbanda and Spiritism traditions. Music and poetry have always nourished me—Tallis, Bach, Shakespeare, Rilke—as well as the great Sufi mystics Rumi, Hafiz, and Sanai, my constant companions.

All these encounters and practices—along with my own quite shattering past-life experiences—have convinced me that there is a reality of the soul to which all mystical phenomena belong. It cannot be proved by science, because it is not a material reality; it is a spiritual reality, accessible only through spiritual and psychological disciplines, such as past-life remembering, that open the gateways to the soul.

As a therapist and teacher who has worked with past-life regression for more than twenty years, I've been asked over and over, "Why bother with past lives? Don't we have enough to worry about in this lifetime?"

Sometimes I play along. "Indeed," I reply, "why bother about the past at all? Why waste so much money on therapy focused on childhood? Surely we're adults now?"

"But that's different," the questioner may say. "Bad things really happened to me in my childhood and they affect me today."

Then I play devil's advocate: "Can you prove they really happened?"

"No, I can't prove it," my questioner says, "but I remember them vividly. In fact, I'd like to forget them."

I take questions like these very seriously, because when I began to be interested in past-life regression, I asked the same questions myself—so much so that my first book on the subject, *Other Lives, Other Selves*, was originally subtitled "A Skeptic Discovers Past Lives." I will do my best to address them in the chapters that follow. But I must emphasize that for me—as for many others—it is not "proof" that convinces, but personal experience.

The experience that convinced me came nearly thirty years ago. I was lying on the sofa when images began to form, at first dimly, then very vividly, and I found myself in 13th-century France, in the thick of the holy war that would come to be called the Albigensian Crusade. I saw the unspeakable horrors of a massacre in a walled city where countless innocents, deemed heretics by the Church, were slaughtered and burned. What was worse, I saw that in the character of a crude mercenary soldier, I was doing the slaughtering myself. I painfully relived an attempted suicide—a leap off a precipice that left me in agony with shattered limbs. I saw my own fearsome death by fire.

A Hollywood re-creation? No movie I have ever seen comes close. Glamorous? By no means. It is a common, clichéd criticism that past-life regressions always turn up Egyptian princesses, Conquistadors, or wives of Henry VIII—prestigious identities to pad a New Age résumé—but my experience held so much shame and violence that I could hardly talk about it. I wanted to disown it, not boast about it. How could this memory be mine? If this was a "past life," I felt, I would do better to keep clear of the subject. Yet as I recovered my soldier's full story and reflected on it more and more (and confirmed the facts in a visit to the hilltop city of Béziers, France, where as many as 20,000 people were massacred in 1208), I came to see how the story explained many things in my life: my inborn fears of fire and heights, a guilt I could never shake, a deep revulsion to most organized religion and militarism, and fragmented images of torture and killing, seen in dreams and meditations over the years, that no amount of psychotherapy had ever really touched.

In the light of these memories—and others, just as vivid—I slowly let go of my prejudices and came to accept, like Hamlet after seeing his father's ghost, that there are more things in heaven and earth than are dreamt of in our philosophy. Since then, I have helped or watched literally thousands of people go through similar experiences—life-changing journeys into psychic memory that help illuminate—and heal—the traumas of the present.

VOYAGES OF TRANSFORMATION

There is no end. There is no beginning.
There is only the infinite passion of life.   —Federico Fellini

Skeptics or believers, those who undergo Deep Memory Process are nearly always moved. The lives they recall tell a vast range of stories, and they are not all Egyptian princesses; they are real people, many of whom could never be identified in history books. They are indigenous people facing invasion, predation, or migration. They are heads of state manipulating great nations. They are feudal lords and genocidal tyrants; emperors, power-mongers, and popes; workers, slaves, and slave masters. They are mothers dying in childbirth, and children lost, enslaved, or sacrificed to the gods. They are victims of every kind of disaster, and survivors of every kind of oppression, whether political, religious, or sexual. They are heroes, cowards, and saints; liberators, benefactors, and martyrs; scheming priestesses, cunning shamans, failed teachers, and dedicated reformers. They are rabble-rousers and camp followers, depressed academics and drunken surgeons, minor poets and mediocre artisans, puritanical judges and professional killers. The list is endless, as is human life.

But in every session, however sad or violent, unfulfilled or unrecognized the past-life self has felt—however frustrated, wasted, or bleak—the rememberer eventually finds himself or herself floating up from the past-life body to know that life is over, that those troubles and wounds can be left behind. He or she has a chance to make a conscious review of the life; to recognize and release patterns (or programs, if you like) that may still be replaying in the present; to forgive or ask forgiveness; and, above all, to seek out lost loved ones or teachers in the world of spirit, where the suffering soul finds healing, wisdom, and peace.

In guiding so many people through the heights and depths of so many lifetimes, and following them on the great crossing into the realms beyond death, I have naturally thought deeply about what takes place on these fantastic voyages into extraordinary visionary spaces—and I have come to question all my assumptions about what memory and imagination really are. Though trained in the Jungian tradition, which values imagination as the language of the soul, I no longer feel that the images we encounter in these regressions are mere images (or even archetypal images), and it no longer helps me to explain them as occurring in some altered state of consciousness. So many of the visions are so vivid, and have such transformative effects on the rememberers, that they seem to speak of other, greater realities than our own.

Slowly, it has dawned on me that when I empathically accompany my clients and students into their inner worlds, following their "imagination" or "memories" on astonishing psychic voyages, I actually move with them into another world: a realm that in many cultures is called the "subtle world," the *mundus imaginalis*, a world real in and of itself. Together, they and I are doing what the shamans call *journeying*, using a highly developed form of imaginative awareness—a visionary capacity closely related to the intuitive sense that psychics and mystics have. I have found, quite simply, that once we cultivate this powerful form of awareness, we can ourselves journey between realities, and directly encounter worlds beyond the physical world, where we have subtle access to the universal source of healing that is Spirit.

IS IT JUST IMAGINATION?

Our culture is used to dismissing anything that does not fit with consensus reality by saying "It's just imagination," which is about the same as saying "You made it up." When someone sees a ghost, people dismiss it as a hallucination; when children see things in the night, parents say, "You're imagining things, go to sleep." In this view imagination is something deceiving, something less than real. Yet the millions of people who pray every day to non-physical beings from Jesus to Mohammed to Lakshmi do so using their "imagination"—their capacity to hold images of the deities in their minds. Is every religious person therefore hallucinating? Do we say that Isaiah, Ezekiel, Saint Teresa, William Blake, and Carl Jung were deluded individuals who "made up" their visions and philosophies? To use *imagination* in such a pejorative, reductive sense is a desecration (literally, "taking out the sacred") of its meaning. Visionary imagination is the most powerful spiritual faculty we have; the power to envision is the capacity that lets us give spiritual shape to both our inner and our outer realities, for good or for ill.

In the Middle Ages, the Scholastics distinguished two types of thinking: *ratio* and *intellectus*. In their view, ratio (usually translated as "reason") belongs to the lower, or reasoning, mind; intellectus (best translated as "intuition" and not to be confused with the modern term *intellect*) belongs to the higher mind that taps into universal truth. A form of spiritual or visionary consciousness, it is the source of all creativity, mystical awareness, and what is sometimes called *gnosis*, or pure knowing. The late British sage and mystic Sir George Trevelyan, whom I was privileged to know, always claimed that these two kinds of thinking corresponded to the two sides of the brain, the left governing the rational functions and the right acting as a conduit to intuitive, mystical knowledge—a direct channel, he would say, to the Divine.

When I talk about imagination here, this is what I mean: not made-up fantasy, but the visionary capacity that is in us all. This capacity is both the language of and the gateway to the soul, transcending time and space to let us access eternal realities only dimly known to our reasoning minds. It has always been available to visionaries, mystics, and charismatics—and regarded by them as a sacred faculty—but for many people it lies dormant until it is awakened. In the chapters that follow and the exercises on the CD, you will find ways to awaken the visionary capacity within you and use it to take your own healing journey into the deep memory of your soul. My purpose is to invite and enable you to make your own exploration and, from what you find, to draw your own conclusions. I cannot offer you proof positive; what I can offer you is stated beautifully by the visionary novelist Hermann Hesse (who was a friend of Jung):

> Only within yourself exists that reality for which you long.
> I can give you nothing that has not already its being within yourself.
> I can throw open to you no picture gallery but your own soul.

CHAPTER ONE

The Story behind the Story

WHEN THERAPY DOES NOT WORK

Many of the problems that we take to our therapists can readily be traced to childhood—events such as losses, abuse, tragedy, and so on—but there are many issues that years of therapy never seem to touch. So many of my clients arrive with deep feelings of grief or with totally inexplicable phobias—a fear of drowning in a boat when they have never been to sea, for instance—that are totally unaccountable in terms of their present life experience. Over and over again, they will remark that they have had such-and-such a feeling ever since they could remember, or that they have always had fantasies about particular countries, or thoughts about certain unpleasant ways of dying, or else strong convictions of having been a different kind of human being in another era.

Such thoughts are by no means to be dismissed. Indeed, the many accumulated cases of past-life remembering from both therapy and research make an almost indisputable case for discarding the scientific dogma (for dogma it is) of the *tabula rasa*—the idea that the mind is a "blank slate" at birth. It is slowly dawning on more and more unprejudiced investigators and common readers that most of our troubles arise from issues we were born with, that the soul has its own history. From this perspective, "past-life therapy," as it has been called for some years, is very much a deep psychology, a psychology of the soul and the deeper tribulations it inherits from the greater history of humanity. As the great French philosopher Michel de Montaigne wrote in his *Essays*: "Each man bears the stamp of the whole human condition."

So when conventional therapy, with its emphasis on our experiences in this life, does not work, the reason may be simple: the therapist is looking for the trauma, the event that caused the psychological disturbance, in the wrong place.

WENDY: A MOTHER'S ANXIETY
"I should never have left them alone!"
One of my clients—a mother I will call Wendy—had terrible anxiety attacks every time she saw her children going off to school or even playing with other children away from the house. She could not bear for them to be away from her for very long, even to go to places like summer camp. She knew that this was unfair, and she did her best to overcome her fears. But as her children got older, the irrational fears remained. She was always anxious about them and called them constantly, even when they were adults with families of their own. She came to see me after a friend brought her own young children over for a visit, because the panic attacks had returned in force—only now someone else's children were triggering Wendy's deep feelings of dread.

Wendy had tried several therapies over the years, but her anxiety had never really gone away. Naturally, she had explored her childhood, but all she had come up with was a terrifying memory of her mother putting her on the school bus when she was about six. Nothing had happened then to account for the fear; it simply appeared that as a little girl, she had been terrified of leaving her home and her mother.

When we probed more deeply in a regression session, we found that in a past life, Wendy had been a Native American boy. In her reliving of the story, the boy went hunting with his father at age ten or eleven, during a time when the tribe was being driven off its land by white men, and came back home to find the family camp on the riverbank under attack. Emerging from the forest, he saw his mother and his younger brother and sister being raped and killed right before his eyes. He and his father rushed down to try to fend the attackers off with knives and bows and arrows, the young boy courageously throwing himself on them, but the white men with their powerful guns mowed them down. The climactic point of the regression came as the boy died, feeling horribly responsible for the death of his family, even though he and his father were actually powerless. His dying thought was, "I should never have left them alone."

Once this story surfaced in Wendy's awareness, it was clear that her childhood fears and her anxiety around her own family had always been unconsciously associated with the Native American boy from the past. Until our session, she had still been afraid that that horror might somehow repeat itself. Just to know that lifetime was an old tape playing in the background of her consciousness was enough to help her erase it and release a great deal of her fear. It sometimes takes further work to break deep habits of fear—but now, at least, Wendy could truthfully tell herself, "My family is safe today. That's just an old story. I can let it go."

SEEKING THE STORY BEHIND THE STORY

We know that many people carry patterns of fear, guilt, and obsessive worry like Wendy's. Clinically, these patterns are labeled "phobias" or "anxiety disorders," yet the psychiatric literature can rarely pinpoint how they arise. What is most puzzling about such feelings is simply that they are irrational; their content does not make sense in and of itself, and there is nothing to connect the fear to our actual life experience. A man who has never been stabbed or badly cut may have a deep fear of knives; a woman who has never sustained a serious burn may have a terrible fear of fire. Casting about in childhood for explanations of such fears does not seem to dislodge them. Often, as in Wendy's case, the problem is already present in childhood, fully formed.

From the perspective of past-life therapy, none of this is surprising: the things we fear—fire, drowning, guns, explosions, savage animals, enclosed spaces, crowds, airplane trips—are not childhood traumas at all, but psychically inherited fears, residues of previous lives still carried deeply in the psychic system we call the unconscious or the soul. The horrors we most fear really happened to someone else, but that "someone else" is still in us today, an imprinted memory from a lifetime that is over, even if the past-life personality does not know it.

When we recognize that irrational fear may come from the experience of another lifetime, then we can search for what I call the "story behind the story"—the old tape, like Wendy's, playing in the background of consciousness. One of Freud's concepts can help us in this regard: the notion of repetition compulsion, which he defined as an uncontrollable urge to replay old behaviors or stories we are no longer conscious of. When we expand this theory beyond a single lifetime, we can quickly see that a person's neurotic behavior, though irrational in the present, may make perfect sense in the context of a story from a past life. The woman with the fear of fire may have been burned at the stake; the man terrified of crowds may have been trampled in a riot; the child frightened of loud noises may remember dying on a battlefield; the adult afraid of flying may have been shot down in a past life as a fighter pilot. Every one of these stories has been recorded in many variations in the annals of past-life regression.

They show us that every complaint—however irrational it seems when isolated as a symptom—can be a clue to a buried story, the soul's way of revealing its most deeply held pain.

CHERYL: FEAR OF THE PUBLIC
Residues of a Roman Lifetime

A very common anxiety is the fear of speaking or appearing in front of a lot of people. This crippling condition can come into play even in small groups, as was the case with my student Cheryl, a young professional psychotherapist who attended one of our workshops on Deep Memory Process. Cheryl was a very able therapist, but she had always suffered from crippling panic attacks when it came to speaking out in public. Until the third day of the workshop, she had successfully avoided such anxiety by deliberately burying her nose in her notebook and saying as little as possible. The topic that morning, however, was fear, and when the talk turned to terror in group situations, she found herself having an anxiety attack at the very mention of the subject. She realized that she needed to talk about what was happening to her, and finally she overcame her fear enough to speak out, albeit with her heart beating fiercely, her palms sweating, and her stomach in knots. The transcript that follows is typical of how we can probe for the "story behind the story"—in this instance, the story behind a story from Cheryl's childhood.

Cheryl It's very difficult for me to say this in front of the group, but I had such a strong flashback a moment ago. I saw myself at a Christmas party in this white dress when I was a little girl. All the family was in the room. I can't go in. I'm terrified. They're all staring at me. And my shoulder is really hurting.

Roger Close your eyes and be back at four years old in your little white dress about to go into the room.

Cheryl (trembling, tearful) I can't. I can't go in. They're all looking down at me. I hate this white dress. Why do they want me to wear it? I'm terrified. Something awful is going to happen. (She sobs deeply.)

Roger (gently helping her focus on the image) Move forward into the room. Go through it. It can't hurt you today.

Cheryl I'm totally frozen. I'm in the room and they're all saying, "What a nice dress. How lovely." I can't look at them. I'm so ashamed and terrified.

Roger What happens?

Cheryl Nothing. I feel better somehow. It's not about them. It was that door, the dress.

Roger Go back again to the most frightening moment, just before you go though the door. That's right. Stay with the fear. Breathe into it. Let the worst image of something awful surface on a count of three. One, two, three!

Cheryl (almost shrieking) Oh, help me, it's a huge crowd. They're screaming at me from above. I'm a grown woman in a white dress. It's Rome. They're going to kill us. Ah! A lion! My arm! I'm not there anymore. I'm above it all looking down. (She has grabbed her arm and bent over in pain. She sobs, then the pain starts to subside and she feels relieved. After many minutes of sobbing, she is finally able to speak.) I saw myself as an early Christian. That was a Roman arena. No wonder I hate white dresses and noisy groups. Thank God that's over.

At the deepest layer of Cheryl's fear, her unconscious mind associated public exposure with a humiliating death. Looking back, we can see that there were several "triggers" here for her. One was being in front of a group—the training group and, earlier, her family. That was the first layer of the story. The second trigger was people looking at her from above, because in the Roman arenas, as we know, the crowd looked down upon the grisly spectacle. The third trigger was the white dress.

What is striking here is that Cheryl's terror initially seemed to arise, as conventional therapy would predict, from a childhood event. Yet remembering her childhood did not reveal the cause of the irrational fear; it merely provided an early example of how the fear was triggered. Clearly, Cheryl's fear of groups came with her at birth, lying dormant until certain situations, like the Christmas party, aroused it. Many of our fears work this way. But there is always a deeper story that will reveal the reason for the soul's debilitating reaction, and when we relive the story, we remove its emotional charge, like a deeply embedded psychic splinter that has always been sensitive when the area around it is touched.

There was another important element in Cheryl's regression experience: the intense shoulder pain, which actually cleared. Such pains, which happen in many regressions, will be discussed further in Chapter 6.

PETER: AN ADOLESCENT'S DEATH WISH
"I'm not going to live very long."

Not all regression journeys need to unpeel a childhood layer of trauma, and not all our stories are about fear. Some problems may lie dormant through childhood, only to be triggered in adolescence or much later in life. My last example of a "story behind the story" is of an angry, disturbed adolescent I will call Peter.

Around the age of seventeen, Peter became very rebellious toward his parents, his teachers, and pretty much anyone around. Familiar adolescent "acting out," we might call it. He got into fights in bars, he drank too much, and when he could get hold of a car, he drove too fast. He actually had a couple of bad motorcycle accidents. To observers, it looked as if he were trying to kill himself. He would probably have denied this; it wasn't at all conscious. But when we probed for the story behind the story, we discovered that he was unconsciously reliving a story in which he was indeed killed. He found himself in a past life as a raw military recruit, pressed into service in the British army. He had been brutalized, sodomized by his superiors, and used as cannon fodder in a horrible battle somewhere in Europe.

In a regression, Peter saw himself as the young soldier, bleeding to death from massive wounds, abandoned to die on the field of the dead. "It's not fair," he groaned. "Why did this happen to me? I never got to live at all. I could have been married, had some kids, run my own little shop somewhere. I hate them, the bastards! Their stupid, meaningless wars. They just use us. They don't give a shit for anything but their own glory. Filthy hypocrites! All that crap about doing it for 'the country.' It's all one big lie!" He could not let go of his hatred and disillusionment with everything the war, and particularly the leaders, stood for. These hugely resentful thoughts became deeply mixed up with all the terror and violence he carried, both in himself and from all the chaos around him as he died. In his despair, the dying soldier took with him the devastating thought that "The world is dangerous and I'm not going to live very long."

This story didn't surface until Peter was an adolescent simply because it had to do with adolescence. In the past life that he was carrying, he had in fact died at around seventeen. All the mindless "acting out" he was doing in the present was a direct consequence of this painfully unfinished past-life story, one that has recurred in my case notes over and over again in numerous variations. But bringing the "story behind the story" to consciousness was a huge relief for Peter. He could now see what was driving him and how he had been living in irrational—but explainable—rage and despair that his life was about to end. He quickly dropped all his self-destructive behaviors and went on to channel his powerful adolescent energies into playing sports and getting into college—both of which he did with great success.

CHAPTER TWO

How We Remember Past Lives

METAPHYSICS AND THE LANGUAGE OF THE SOUL

Science can help us grasp the profound mysteries of the material universe, but if we truly want to understand the mysteries of memory, imagination, and visionary experience—including past-life memory—we will have to go beyond conventional scientific thinking. Interestingly, the Greek word for "beyond" is *meta*. We are all familiar with at least the title of Aristotle's *Metaphysics*, the book the great Greek philosopher wrote after the *Physics* to go beyond the study of the purely material world.

So when we talk about past-life memories, we need to be aware that they are not simply emanations of the physical realm, but that they derive from higher or subtle realities. When the poet Wordsworth says that "trailing clouds of glory do we come from God, who is our home," his striking poetic language reminds us that the consciousness of the newborn child is a luminous consciousness, one that carries the imprint of this subtle reality, the reality of the soul. We find the same idea in traditions such as astrology, which claims that when a child is born (or conceived, in Chinese astrology), the agendas of the soul are already imprinted. This has nothing to do with physiology or genetics. It is the imprinting of psychically determined patterns coming from a higher level of reality, the non-material vibrational frequency (to borrow a metaphor from science) that belongs to higher mind.

Aristotle openly acknowledged, following his great mentor Plato, that there was another level to be studied, one beyond, above, and higher than the physical. Notice that all these metaphors have spatial connotations. They suggest a different kind of space: psychic space, that is to say, spiritual reality. But to access higher realities—and our own higher minds—we do not need to climb a ladder or perform brain surgery; instead, we need to alter our state of consciousness. For the simple truth is that it is by directing our awareness inward in a quiet, meditative way, toward the vast psychic realm of dream image, memory, and vision that we each carry, that we are able to encounter these other realities.

Transpersonal psychology also reminds us that, in order to talk about the transcendent reality through which higher consciousness and past-life memories are transmitted to us, we have to distinguish between different levels of the personality. In other words, we will need to speak not just of an ordinary day-to-day self but of a higher self as well. And there are plenty of precedents for this in sacred tradition and esoteric literature.

From the perspective of earthly life, it is common to refer to the self that deals with day-to-day reality as the *ego* or *ego personality*. This ego develops from infancy to adulthood to become our *biographical self*. Its thoughts, feelings, memories, and perceptions are the subject of conventional psychology, the study of what we call our *personality*. But to talk of dimensions that transcend the physical world—of encounters with states where people experience mystical raptures, cosmic consciousness, and shamanic journeys to other worlds—transpersonal psychology rightly proposes the existence of a self-aware consciousness, a greater or a higher Self.

OPENING THE "HEAVENLY EYE"

When our consciousness is altered or expanded through the cultivation of meditative, visionary, or trance states, we are much more in touch with this greater Self and its higher, more lucid awareness. If we transcend the material, one-dimensional perceptions of our this-worldly ego personalities, we are able to become aware of realities far beyond physical reality; we learn to see in a way that the ancients called *sub specie aeternitatis*, which means "from the eye or perspective of eternity."

In the writings of early Buddhism, we find a sermon in which the Buddha says something very similar:

With the heavenly eye purified and beyond range of human vision, I saw how beings vanish and come to be again. I saw high and low, brilliant and insignificant, and how each attained, according to his karma, a favorable or a painful birth.

This subtle vision is not nearly as difficult to acquire as one might think. Many of us are already familiar with it through working with our dreams; in fact, it is the same consciousness that is with us in the dream state, particularly if we have developed it to the degree of lucid dreaming. Throughout this book, you will have opportunities to develop your own "heavenly eye," along with the other subtle senses that are available to us in meditative or visionary states of consciousness.

The key to opening the heavenly eye is learning to work with images, developing our capacity to imagine vividly and deeply. And imaging does not always mean visualizing. Some of us hear images; we have a more auditory imagination than others. Some of us feel or sense images; we know what it is like to be in a certain place physically, to sense the environment, to feel a different body. Playwrights and filmmakers, for example, are often highly intuitive with their physical images; they can set scenes in their imagination with incredible precision before realizing them on stage or film. But everyone imagines in a slightly different way. If our visual images are not clear, we may have strong kinesthetic or physical images instead.

IMAGINATION: A BRIDGE TO THE SUBTLE REALMS

I believe that in its higher form (as opposed to fantasy, its lower or ego-related form), imagination is the bridge to the transpersonal realities of the soul, that transcendent part of the personality we have called the *Self*. This level of reality is also called the *subtle world* or the *spirit world*. Platonism, Hinduism, and Buddhism, all of which subscribe to the idea of the transmigration of the soul, call it the *intermediary world*, a reality midway between this world and the world of pure light. (In Tibetan Buddhism, this in-between place is called a *bardo*.) This measureless, infinite world beyond the material world is the source not only of all the memories and experiences of humanity, but also of all dreams and visions. In the Hindu tradition, this is thought to be a universal cosmic substrate or subtle vibrational field, called the *akasha*, that runs through and underlies every form or event in time and space, whether material or psychic. (Edgar Cayce, a medium who read past lives, talked of the *akashic record*.) The scholar Joseph Campbell called it *mythic reality*. The Aborigines in Australia call it the *dreamtime*.

The dreamtime remains largely a mystery to us in the modern world because as a culture we have not taken it seriously for a long time. We are too caught up with the material world to notice it, except in states of distraction or retreat. And yet it is always there, always waiting to be visited. We can go into it like Alice in Wonderland, through the rabbit hole, as in shamanic journeying, or we can cross the bridge of imagination. (In fact, in visionary geography, most journeys into the other realm do require a formal crossing or rite of passage: a tunnel, a door-way, a corridor, a bridge, a window, or a portal opening to the other side.)

TRAVELING IN VISIONARY TIME AND SPACE

As a little test of your ability to imagine, I reproduce a short poem from an English poet, Robert Graves, called "Warning to Children." It is addressed to the playful and curious child in each of us whose imagination has not been entirely stifled by too much rational education:

Children, if you dare to think
Of the greatness, rareness, muchness
Fewness of this precious only
Endless world in which you say
You live, you think of things like this:
Blocks of slate enclosing dappled
Red and green, enclosing tawny
Yellow nets, enclosing white
And black acres of dominoes,
Where a neat brown paper parcel
Tempts you to untie the string.
In the parcel a small island,
On the island a large tree,
On the tree a husky fruit.

Strip the husk and pare the rind off:
In the kernel you will see
Blocks of slate enclosed by dappled
Red and green, enclosed by tawny
Yellow nets, enclosed by white
And black acres of dominoes,
Where the same brown paper parcel—
Children, leave the string alone!
For who dares undo the parcel
Finds himself at once inside it,
On the island, in the fruit,
Blocks of slate about his head,
Finds himself enclosed by dappled
Green and red, enclosed by yellow
Tawny nets, enclosed by black
And white acres of dominoes,
With the same brown paper parcel
Still untied upon his knee.
And, if he then should dare to think
Of the fewness, muchness, rareness,
Greatness of this endless only
Precious world in which he says
he lives—he then unties the string.

As you read the poem, notice how quickly you move through realities in your imaging, how you move from parcel to island to tree to fruit and back again in split seconds. In the imagination, we can go anywhere, be in any place instantly.

That is not to say we are going there physically, but traveling in that "other" world that mirrors this one. According to the Sufi philosopher Al Ghazzali, the higher world is a spiritual image of the lower world, so that when we travel in the visionary or imaginary realm, we are actually moving in another reality.

This is precisely what happens in past-life journeying. When we tap into the vast memory store that is both ours and all humankind's, we can move anywhere in human history instantly. It is not a slow, laborious process at all; it is no different from remembering events in this life. If I ask you, "Do you remember last Christmas?" you can call up images instantly, almost as soon as I suggest them. If I say, "Think of the house you grew up in," the image is there at once. Our power of recall operates a bit like a computer—we can call up these memory programs just by naming them. Every image has a name attached to it, and vice versa. If you can name something with words, you can call up an image of it.

CD TRACK I

A Memory Exercise: Re-Imagining Childhood Games

At this point, you may be ready to begin training yourself in the art of memory and imagination. For most of us, a good place to start is our childhood, where our sense of play and our affinity for fantasy were especially strong.

In this exercise, you will be guided to free-associate back into your childhood and to re-imagine all kinds of things you once did or experienced, but may well have forgotten. You will be surprised how vividly all sorts of events surface, quite spontaneously, once you just let go and follow the stream of images that comes. It does not matter whether it is fantasy or memory. What is most important is to get into a playful frame of mind and let your "inner child" take over for the space of the exercise.

Headphones are excellent for this type of exercise. Have available a notebook, a pen, and drawing paper and crayons in case you feel inspired after the exercise to record the memories or draw the images that emerge. Now find a quiet place where you will not be disturbed, and listen to Track 1 of the enclosed CD.

A NOTE ON THE FIRST MEMORY EXERCISE

As you work through this exercise, you may find yourself in a simple, happy scene: perhaps working in a garden, looking after children, working as a merchant, or reliving a scene from another childhood in a past life. But you may also meet resistance or touch on troubling scenes. When we challenge the unconscious mind, when we try to go in deeply, we sometimes "block"—it is as though the images freeze up and we cannot go anywhere—and this is usually because the story that is coming to mind has unpleasant associations. There may be sadness involved. There may be loss. In past lifetimes, as in the present, just as many tragedies happen in childhood as in adulthood—and trauma makes a deeper impression on a young child than on an adult. So do not be surprised if you find yourself having strong emotions or feeling a little confused when you start to do this exercise and the ones that follow.

I often say that when we open the door to past-life memory, half a dozen major lifetimes will want to surface to begin with. It does not matter, in my experience, which exercise or which technique we use to get at them; the same stories will be there. In fact, when you first break into a past lifetime, it is often that one and that one alone that will come up in subsequent regressions. It is as though you cannot move on to the next lifetime until you have fully explored the one at hand. ✎

CHAPTER
THREE

Past Lives,
Present Problems

GETTING TRIGGERED

In the last chapter and CD exercise, you were guided to call up images from your childhood and then free-associate to images from a past life. You may have seen some vivid but essentially peaceful scenes from another lifetime. But it is possible that some strong feelings, such as sadness or fear, also arose. You may even have come upon an upsetting scene you preferred not to look at. Or maybe you blocked altogether.

All these reactions are common, and it is impossible to predict how any individual will react when delving into the past-life memory banks; we have to risk the experiment. But when you do have a strong reaction—especially blocking—chances are you are being "triggered." Very often, the portal into a past-life memory is a distressing event in our present life that awakens, or triggers, an older or deeper memory. In the examples we explored in Chapter 1—Wendy's story of the Indian raid, Cheryl's fear from the Roman arena, and

Peter's adolescent death wish—we saw how events in each of their lives had caused emotional chaos for many years. But we also saw how paying precise attention to the triggering situation in the present could open the door to the past. What follows is the story of a young woman who walked through just such a door.

SALLY: THE DEAD CHILD
"It was all my fault."

This woman, whom I will call Sally, was living on the coast of California and training in massage at a school in Big Sur. She was in her thirties and had lived a fairly solitary life with few close relationships. She later admitted that she had never wanted to have a family in this lifetime.

Sally was driving back from San Francisco to Big Sur when she came upon a terrible car accident. A car had gone off the side of the road, rolled down the mountainside, and become wedged in the rocks. Several people had stopped their cars and were looking on in horror. Someone had called the state police.

Sally, who had a degree in nursing and basic first-aid knowledge, was a practical type, so she scrambled down the cliff and tried to get into the car. Inside, there was the body of a woman, clearly dead. Now, the interesting thing is that the sight of the dead woman did not upset Sally in any way, but when she looked around to see if there was anyone else in the car or beside the car, she saw something that did affect her—a baby bottle. It was at that point that she lost control—"freaked out," as she put it—and started to tremble and weep. She was so overcome that she did not look for the body of the baby, but just scrambled back up the rocks to get away. She said to the state trooper, "There's a dead woman down there, and I think a baby, you take over, I can't do anything." Then she got into her car and drove, trembling, all the way home.

That memory was still with her three weeks later, when Sally came to a workshop. I asked her to focus on that moment when she saw the baby bottle and "freaked out." I said, "What does that baby bottle make you think of?"

"I was too late," she said.

I said gently, "Go on!"

"I was too late to save the baby."

"Repeat that phrase a few times and see where it takes you."

"It's too late, it's too late," she said. "Oh, my God, the baby's dead."

"Where are you?" I asked her.

Sally saw herself on a mountainside in Scotland. She immediately felt that she had the stocky body of a Scottish peasant woman. She was up tending the sheep, and she had heard gunfire from the little village where she lived. It was the seventeenth century, when there were violent skirmishes between the English and the Scottish border people. She came running down the hill, burst into her cottage, and found her sister and two babies—her own and her sister's—all shot, all dead. "I was too late," she said. "I should have been there for my child. It was all my fault."

Just the thought of a dead baby had taken Sally through a doorway into another lifetime. Once I invited her to focus, the transition was almost instant. When she was first triggered, she was too upset to stay with the process and examine the images, but they were right there, close to the surface. It simply took a step through that doorway to find herself in another lifetime. It was a painful life to remember, but it helped her understand why in this lifetime she had chosen not to have children. By the time our sessions together were over, she was able to forgive herself for the failure in her past life, and look more favorably at relationships, and even consider the possibility of a family.

Sally's story is similar in many ways to Wendy's memory of the Native American boy who could not save his family from the killing; indeed, such stories must have been repeated thousands of times in our bloody colonial history. But the Scottish woman, as the mother of the child, was left with different, though equally devastating, feelings; she blamed herself for not saving the baby, a guilt only a mother could feel. So although the Scottish woman died peacefully in her bed in that life, the memory of that terrible day stayed with her and went with her into the subtle realm after death, to be retransmitted as one of Sally's soul wounds today. At some level, though she never fully verbalized it to herself, Sally thought she would not be a good mother. No matter how good she might actually be with kids—and it was clear from her massage work that she was a very nurturing woman—such half-expressed thoughts totally undermined her self-worth until they were brought to consciousness and their roots rendered harmless.

OUR COMPLEXES, OUR KARMA

As Carl Jung once observed, everyone knows we have complexes; what we forget is that complexes "have" us! The powerful past-life stories behind the present-day problems of Wendy and the others are just that—complexes, but not complexes formed in childhood, as the Freudians would have it; rather, complexes built around the deeper memories that belong to the soul. So it is no exaggeration to say that our karmic wounds from the distant past become the complexes of the present.

In every past-life complex ever studied, there lies frozen or buried a strong emotion or feeling (fear, shame, guilt, pride, rage); a buried thought or assumption ("I can never do enough," "I have to do it alone," "They'll all laugh at me"); often a bodily pain (headache, sexual block, skin rash, bowel problems); and always fragments of a script or story (victim of a witch-hunt, betrayal in the senate, the tribe wiped out). In the table below, you will see how broad a range of complexes past-life therapy can uncover, and the typical stories behind each one.

PAST-LIFE COMPLEXES: COMMON THEMES AND STORIES

- **Insecurity and fear of abandonment.** Often related to past-life memories of literal abandonment: being orphaned, sold into slavery, left out to die in times of famine, separated from loved ones during a crisis or a war, etc.
- **Depression and low energy.** Loss of a loved one or a parent; unfinished grieving; suicide memories; despair as a result of war, massacre, imprisonment, or deportation.
- **Phobias and irrational fears.** May be caused by all kinds of trauma in a past life: death by fire, water, suffocation, animals, knives, insects, natural disasters.
- **Sadomasochistic behavior problems.** Usually related to a past-life memory of torture, often with loss of consciousness, usually with sexual overtones. The pain and rage seem to perpetuate hatred and a desire to revenge oneself in the same way.
- **Guilt and martyr complexes.** Commonly stem from past-life memories of killing a loved one, sacrificing a child, ordering the deaths of others, or feeling responsible for their deaths (e.g., in a fire). The entrenched thought is most often, "It's all my fault. I deserve this."
- **Material insecurity and eating disorders.** Past-life memories of starvation, economic collapse, or inescapable poverty; may manifest as anorexia, bulimia, or obesity.
- **Accidents, violence, physical brutality.** Repetition of battlefield memories from warrior lives; unfulfilled quests for power; love of adventure. This complex is common in adolescence, the time of life when many soldiers historically met their deaths.

- **Family struggles.** Past-life scores to settle with parents, children, or siblings: betrayal, abuse of power, inheritance injustices, rivalries. Includes most Oedipal dynamics.
- **Sexual difficulties and abuse.** Problems of frigidity, impotence, and genital infection often have past-life stories of rape, abuse, or torture behind them. Even cases of incest and abuse may turn out to be reruns of past-life patterns where emotional release was blocked.
- **Marital difficulties.** These sometimes derive from past lives with the same mate in a different power, class, or sexual constellation: e.g., as master, mistress, slave, prostitute, or concubine, or where the sex roles were reversed.
- **Chronic physical ailments.** Reliving of traumatic injuries or deaths. Headaches may relate to intolerable mental choices in other lives; throat ailments to verbal denunciations or unspoken thoughts; ulcers to memories of terror; neck-aches to hanging and strangling. Therapy often relieves chronic pain in these areas.

Source: Roger J. Woolger, *Other Lives, Other Selves* (Doubleday, 1987)

The healing work of past-life therapy is therefore fourfold:

1. To thaw the old, frozen feelings and release blocked energy
2. To bring negative thoughts and assumptions into consciousness in order to recognize their origins, see that they no longer belong to our current life, and let them go so we can then replace them with more positive, life-affirming thoughts
3. To release pains or blocks held in the body (more on this in Chapter 6)

4. To replay the old story and bring about a resolution in the mind of the past-life character

In most cases, the most effective starting point is to relive the story as realistically as possible. Therapists have always known the power of role-playing to unlock our complexes; in past-life work, reliving creates a kind of psychodrama that in and of itself offers opportunities to release blocked emotions. The psychodramatic approach also enables us to detach from negative thoughts by seeing how they belong to an old and essentially outworn drama. We find we have been living a long-ago nightmare that no longer needs to have power over us. And a complex that no longer "has" us has lost its charge; its energy can now be used more creatively.

Few emotions carry such strong charges as anger and rage—but at the same time, nothing can be as devastating as holding these feelings in. Since the early twentieth century, the bodywork of Reich has observed the dire energetic effects of holding suppressed rage deeply in the body; more recently, therapists have developed "rage reduction" workshops to discharge toxic anger. Even so, not all therapists are comfortable helping release rage, and some prefer to avoid it. But past-life therapy has found that remembering the source of old rage and expressing it within the psychodramatic context of the past-life story can be enormously effective, as well as satisfying to the person who releases the pent-up violence from his or her system. Release such as this was first given a name by Aristotle, who observed the powerful effects of emotion on audiences in the theaters of ancient Greece: weeping and moaning in anguish as they identified with the sufferings of Orestes or Oedipus, they experienced a kind of emotional purgation, a cleansing—in short, a *catharsis*.

ELMORE: DEPRESSION AND BACK PAIN
A Slave's Old Hatred

An African-American named Elmore came to a workshop to explore the depressions he had suffered throughout his adult life. As a psychiatrist, he had taken various medications for relief over the years, but the symptoms never fully went away. In talking about himself, he also mentioned recurrent back pain that had troubled him for a long time.

When he went into a past-life regression, he found himself as a powerfully built slave on a sugar plantation. He was a bitter and rebellious slave who ran away on several occasions. He was always plotting how to get out. But each time, he was caught, brought back, and savagely beaten, typically on the back. Finally, after the fifth or sixth attempt, his masters were so angry that they beat him to death, his back taking most of the punishment.

Elmore relived the death of the slave in a psychodrama, assisted by other workshop members: his arms were lightly tied in a towel to suggest the struggle in his body, and he was whipped, but very gently, to suggest the beating. The effect was obvious to observers as he tensed his back, held his breath, and clenched his teeth. Naturally, the slave was holding tremendous rage in his back and arms. Because he could not express it, he took it with him at death, everything frozen into those tense areas of his back, chest, arms, and respiratory system. His dying thoughts, clenched in his body, were, "It's hopeless. There's nothing I can do. I'll never be free. I hate them. I could kill them."

I encouraged Elmore to go through the death and remember exactly what it was like. Once it was over, he reported those feelings of enormous frustration and the tension remaining in his back. But above all, he was left with despair and hopelessness because he was so powerless to fight back. It was clear that the slave had died with intense feeling lodged in his back and other parts of his body, but they were frozen, still clenched with rage and pain.

The story seemed so unresolved, emotionally and physically, that I asked Elmore: "If you could have fought these masters back, what would you have done?" He said, "I would have beaten them back, I would have thrown them off me and beaten them back." Above all, he wanted to use his elbows to get them literally off his back. So, in a second cathartic psychodrama, I gave him some thick cushions and encouraged him to show us what that rage would look like if he dramatized it physically. I gave him plenty of space, and he beat up the cushions with obvious relish, making a lot of noise in the process and breathing hard and emotionally. In a very powerful catharsis, he was able to release the rage of a powerless slave that he had carried in his body all his life.

When Elmore reflected on the experience, he saw clearly that his work as a psychiatrist in a hospital—because of the power structure there—had made him feel powerless and constantly resentful. He recognized that he had actually felt powerless all his life and that he had always put himself in work situations in institutional hierarchies where he felt he was under someone else's thumb. Even though he had a strong personality, he never fought back and he never challenged authority. It was clear to him now how he had carried those feelings of power-lessness and rage with him from the slave life; he saw that the despair he had felt then was a perfect mirror of his depressions today. He even admitted that he felt trapped in his job and that his inability to leave it was depressing him. Clearly, his job situation had been an ongoing trigger for him, and because he never expressed these feelings, they had turned to poison in his system and contributed a great deal to his emotional and physical pain.

CD TRACK 2
Exploring Personal Difficulties: An Emotional Release Exercise
This exercise is designed to help you use an issue that causes personal difficulty

in your life today as a bridge to reach the deeper unconscious, where your past-life memories are stored. It will help you probe one of the emotional patterns that you may be stuck in or an attitude that is somehow limiting you. First, you will focus on your personal experience and memories of when this issue has been troublesome to you. Then, as you did in the first exercise, you will be gently invited to keep going deeper into different layers of your memory. By just allowing yourself to free-associate, exactly as you did in the first exercise, you will find that similar images and feelings will start to surface from a past-life scenario. Simply let anything surface of its own accord, and quietly ignore any skeptical or critical thoughts that may want to interfere. You will not need to reproduce a whole lifetime, but simply focus on a particularly strong scene and release the charge in it.

As you did for the first exercise, use headphones if you like. Again, have available a notebook, paper, and crayons to draw with in case you feel inspired after the exercise to record your images and memories. For this exercise, it is also a good idea to have handy a towel to twist, a pillow to hit, and some tissues for any tears that the work might provoke. Now find a quiet place where you will not be disturbed, and listen to Track 2 of the enclosed CD.

CHAPTER FOUR

The Soul's
Unfinished Business

Zen has no other secrets than seriously thinking about birth-and-death.
—Takeda Shingen

He who dies before he dies, does not die when he dies.
—Abraham of Santa Clara

WORKING WITH THE STORY BEHIND THE STORY

The value of remembering past lifetimes is frequently that feelings long buried or blocked can come to the surface and be released. Old fears, as we have seen, can be re-run and found to be baseless: we find that they no longer apply today, that they are simply old stories somehow lodged into the psyche. Generally speaking, it is in lifetimes where there were traumas and severe struggle, or where the life span was cut short, that phobic or traumatic patterns are most likely to be passed on. One of the meanings of the word *karma* is actually "work"; in contemporary usage I often translate it simply as "the soul's unfinished business." The things we failed to do, the setbacks we experienced in one lifetime, seem to be passed on as the soul's ongoing tasks—work to be redone by the newly incarnating consciousness as it returns to this world in new circumstances and with new opportunities.

REPLAYING PAST-LIFE SCRIPTS

We have seen how old stories, carried quite unconsciously, can become the driving force behind the continuous scripts and compulsive patterns that dominate our current lives. We find ourselves attracting misfortunes, bad relationships, or persistent unhappiness. We all know people, for example, who go from one bad relationship to another, always replaying the same betrayal script; we all know people who are chronically accident-prone.

I was once consulted by a client who had lived with an endless stream of physical accidents, broken bones, and seeming bad luck. Her friends would no longer drive with her because she had been in so many car accidents. When she explored her problem in a regression, she saw herself in a past life as a Polynesian woman about to be crushed by an enormous tidal wave. As the water engulfed her entire village, her terrified dying thought, frozen in her, was, "I'll never get away from this. It's going to hit me." Sure enough, throughout her present life, things kept hitting her: cars and horses and large objects. Only when she let go of the Polynesian woman's terror did the accidents stop.

Such dire karmic scripts can almost always be traced to some personal tragedy, trauma, or cataclysm in a past life: The loss of those we love. Our possessions destroyed in upheaval or war. Suffering deportation or imprisonment. Being orphaned as a child. Dying of starvation on the street. Invasion, rape, enslavement—they only scratch the surface of "the thousand natural shocks that flesh is heir to," in the famous words of Shakespeare's Hamlet. Traumas like these deeply disturb the equilibrium of the soul, leaving parts of it emotionally frozen. They create patterns of suffering that in Sanskrit are called *samskaras*—deep and bitter scars in the soul that carry over from lifetime to lifetime. Few of us can escape the heritage of psychic scars from emotional and material loss, violence, abuse, abandonment, betrayal, or scapegoating in one lifetime or another. These wounds, rarely healed in the lifetime when they occurred, return, alas, "as instruments to plague us," as Shakespeare wrote in

King Lear, his most devastating play (and one in which karma plays a key part). He also wrote of how the samskaras return with us at birth:

We came crying hither;
Thou know'st the first time that we smell the air
We waul and cry.

So it is no surprise that our first examples—the attack on the Native American camp, the flashback to the Roman arena, and the battlefield—all involved sudden and violent death. Human history is full of invasions, massacres, and atrocities related to times of war and upheaval, and more often than not, past-life stories do involve untimely death. None of these stories is pleasant, and few are heroic, but the violent ones need to be rooted out much as a dentist extracts a rotten tooth. In this chapter, we will look more closely at past-life scars left by premature death in war, violence, and catastrophe, and we will see how careful attention can release their hold on us today.

WHERE THE SOUL GOES AFTER DEATH

We understand death, transition, and rebirth more deeply today than ever, thanks to valuable work in a wide range of traditions. In hospitals, the work of the hospice movement has helped us break the habit of denial and learn to give death its due; the writings of pioneers like Raymond Moody, Kenneth Ring, and Elisabeth Kübler-Ross have given us a remarkable glimpse of what awaits on the other side. In these powerful accounts of near-death experiences, people who have clinically died but returned to tell the tale report passing through tunnels to a world of light, where they may have deeply moving reviews of their life on earth, meet spirits of ancestors and other luminous beings, or find themselves guided on awesome trips around the cosmos. Finally, they return to their bodies, usually with great pain, but with their beliefs, their consciousness, and their attitudes to life and death transformed forever. Accounts of past-life regression—including those in my own files—chart strikingly similar experiences of passing beyond death, reviewing one's life, meeting spirits and guides, and journeying into other dimensions.

After conducting or observing many, many regressions, I have noted that there are roughly three states the departing spirit or soul may find itself in as it leaves the body:

- **Earthbound** The departing spirit stays stuck on earth, either fixed or wandering, unaware that its earthly life has ended.
- **Unfinished or troubled:** The spirit moves to a higher after-death realm, but in a state of confusion, still obsessed with the life just ended; if this confusion does not clear (and it often does not), it is recycled into a subsequent rebirth.
- **Completed or enlightened** The spirit is fully freed from the dross of earthly memories and goes peacefully to an even higher plane, a pure realm of light.

The greater part of the work I do as a therapist working with past lives naturally concerns the first two of these categories, simply because the traumatic and tragic stories, with their fears, failures, and "stuck-ness," most clearly show us exactly where and how deeply karmic patterns were established, and how they still trouble us today. Your own regression work, using the exercises on the CD, concerns the second category, as you examine your transitions between lives and the complexes you have carried with you into the present.

To deepen our understanding of the soul's transition still further, we can look to the wisdom of the Tibetan Buddhist tradition and its teachers in the West. Forty years ago, only scholars of Buddhism (and Carl Jung!) knew much about the *Bardo Thodol*, or *Tibetan Book of the Dead*, with its explicit instructions to the soul upon leaving the body at death. Today we have Sogyal Rinpoche's *Tibetan Book of Living and Dying*, a superb amplification of the ancient text, in which he explains its archaic symbols in modern psychospiritual language to demystify the stages of consciousness that the psyche passes through after death.

In the Tibetan view, the after-death realm—called a *bardo* (literally, "the in-between"), an intermediary realm in between lifetimes—is a real place. Tibetan tradition teaches that when the spirit leaves the body, it spends a time in this intermediary realm and goes through a series of experiences, partly to help it let go of the lifetime that has passed and partly to prepare it, ideally, for becoming "completed" or "enlightened" and leaving the earth plane altogether. The spirit may be faced with beings, entities, or energies that mirror the unfinished psychological problems of the person who has died. Unless the dying consciousness can assimilate these difficult forces it encounters, it is reborn and sent back to earth. What is extraordinary about the Tibetan teachings is the way in which the consciousness after death is treated as a fully human consciousness, essentially the same as it was when in a body on earth. Sogyal Rinpoche sums it up in one remarkable statement: "Tibetan Buddhism has left us the still revolutionary insight that birth and death are both in the mind and nowhere else." Ultimately, whether you are in a body or out of a body, mind is continuous.

Birth and death, then, are part of a profound, continuous cycle. The extraordinary work of psychologist Stanislav Grof and others on intrauterine regression reveals that, as the fetus gets closer to the moment of birth and the compression that takes place in the uterus gets stronger, dark and painful memories are stimulated: memories of dismemberment, crucifixion, burning, crushing, and all kinds of horrible death. The birth canal itself is a mirror image of the tunnel that the soul travels through when it leaves the body. Coming back into the body is a reverse tunnel, and a painful one. In my book *Other Lives, Other Selves*, I have suggested that death, birth, and the realm between form a kind of loop that we go through; the way we come in often mirrors the way we died in a previous lifetime. To take the simplest example: a person born with the umbilical cord wrapped around his neck may, when regressed spontaneously, remember how, in a previous lifetime, he was hanged.

OUR DYING THOUGHTS

In the most common regression experience of dying in a past life—whether in a peaceful or a violent death—the rememberer finds himself or herself leaving the body and simply floating upward. Sometimes the departed spirit hovers over the body, taking in the fact that it is all over; it may stay looking down over the body until the body is buried or cremated. But unlike an "earthbound" spirit, this departed spirit is consciously aware of having died, and this awareness frees the soul to travel up into the higher dimensions of the bardo. The transition can actually be quite beautiful: one sees the earth from above, is shown a panoramic visionary overview of one's life, and may be shown the progress of loved ones left on earth. Eventually, there is a feeling of having arrived in another dimension, another realm.

But if the circumstances of death have been at all difficult, or if the person was emotionally disturbed in any way before death—resentful, vengeful, guilty, lonely, or fearful, for instance—it is the intensity of those emotions and corresponding thoughts that will go with the departing spirit, obscuring the potentially uplifting and reassuring aspects of the transition. Some years ago, I was struck by a comment W. Evans-Wentz made in his famous early translation of *The Tibetan Book of the Dead*: "Buddhists and Hindus alike believe that the last thought at the moment of death determines the character of the next incarnation." From then on, I started to look very carefully during regression work at what people were going through as they were dying in a past life. I found that the death experience and the way people clung to life—dying angry, or bitter, or with despairing thoughts—said a great deal about their attitudes toward living in their current lives.

Typical thoughts and feelings that occur at the moment of death have now been recorded from thousands of regressions. "They didn't want me," "They didn't care about me," are the thoughts of children who had been put out to die or get lost in some kind of attack. "I have to do it all alone," "There's no one to help me," say people who are left to struggle and die alone. People who died in a famine say that "There wasn't enough, there was never enough." People who were killed for speaking out or crossing some line say, "I should have kept silent," "I should have kept it to myself." Others feel guilty: "I could have done more," "It's all my fault," "I didn't do enough." Thoughts may be vengeful: "I'll get back at them," "I'll hurt them the way they hurt me." We may have negative thoughts about ourselves—"I'm no good," "I was useless," "I didn't help them," "I failed them"—or about some physical failure: "I'll never walk again," "I'm trapped," "I'll never get out of this." Someone forced into degrading sexual behavior may say, "I'm disgusting." Someone who has been betrayed may say, "I'll never trust anyone again," "It's not safe to show what I really feel," "People will let you down," "It's all lies." When people have died in despair or resigned to hopeless situations such as incarceration or slavery, we hear thoughts that will sow the seeds of depression and negativity

in future incarnation: "Why bother to do anything?" "What's the use?" "They always win." "It'll never change."

MADELINE: CHRONIC PAIN
A Reminder of Past Brutality

A particularly devastating kind of dying thought, one that we meet not infrequently in past-life death scenarios, has to do with guilt and self-hatred. A woman whom I will call Madeline had suffered for much of her life from severe pain in her neck and shoulder area. She had done all kinds of bodywork, but the pain never quite went away. She herself was a social worker whose charges were children with learning deficiencies. She was an extremely gentle woman and was very concerned with her clients. But in the past-life story she uncovered, she was a slave owner who had brutalized so many slaves that one day a group of them decided to take their revenge. They ganged up on the master, hid behind a building, and, when he emerged, grabbed him and beat him to death. The final, fatal blow was a blow to the neck.

As the slave owner died, he realized very clearly what was going on, how much rage was directed at him, and his dying thought was, "I treated them brutally. These are my just deserts." When he found himself leaving his body and looking down at it, still being beaten by the angry slaves, he took these thoughts with him: "I shouldn't have treated human beings in that way. I deserve to be punished." Not surprisingly, it was the neck and shoulders where the slave owner "took the punishment" and where the residues of the old pain re-imprinted themselves in Madeline's body. Immediately, Madeline recognized why she had been carrying this pain in her neck all her life—the physical imprint of the slave owner's guilt. She was still blaming herself by replaying the old violence against her body. And she was still working in this lifetime to make up for the slave owner's evil ways by working with children in need of help. Once she could see all of this, and once she was able to help the old slave owner within her talk to the slaves and ask their forgiveness, she felt a huge unburdening of the guilt and the pain.

SARAH: A LOST BROTHER AND THE NAZIS
"I'll come and find you."

Dying thoughts from a past life can have much happier consequences in the present than Madeline's persistent neck pain. A different kind of unfinished business came to light when my client Sarah uncovered her past life as an adolescent Jewish girl in the Second World War. She saw herself reliving the horrors that her small Polish village endured when the community suddenly fell victim to the Nazis. In the chaos, she and her mother tried to hide while her father and older brother, to whom she was deeply attached, fled to the woods with other men to try to form some kind of resistance to the Nazi occupation, but there was no time for the young girl and her other siblings to escape. They were dragged out of hiding, many of them raped, some shot; most of the women and children and elderly were eventually herded into cattle trucks and shipped to the concentration camps.

The parting words from her older brother rang in her ears as he headed for the woods: "I'll come and find you." But that was the last she heard of him. Eventually she died in the camp, thinking as she went to the gas chamber, "I want to be with my brother. I wish he had come back." Then, in her present lifetime, Sarah found herself very strongly attracted to a colleague who was married and had his own family (just as she does in this life). She started to work with this colleague; they even formed their own business. They felt incredibly close. And when she finally did her regression, she recognized that this colleague was none other than the brother she had been seeking from that past life. They had indeed found each other; such was the power of those parting and dying thoughts.

RIGHT LIVING, RIGHT DYING

At the heart of these unfinished thoughts at death are the most primal of human passions. Raw recruits may still be bitter; they died too young on the battlefield; they are angry with the people who condemned them to a worthless death. Others feel profound grief at leaving behind loved ones, regret at not having done more. Obsessive thoughts of revenge may drive the soul back into another incarnation to finish what was started. Although most accounts of near-death experience suggest an automatic review of the lifetime just ended, this is not always the case in past-life death scenarios, for if the feelings of revenge are too strong, they may catapult the soul straight into rebirth, bypassing any chance for reflection. Equally obsessive in their way are dying thoughts like Sarah's, or those of a mother who has lost her son in a massacre and then dies herself, thinking, "I've got to find him; I've got to be with him." A thought this determined—"I've got to find him"—inevitably means that her soul will follow the soul of her son very quickly into another life-time, often with no time to review her last life in the realm between lives.

In the next chapter, we will consider in more detail the many scenarios and encounters that occur between lifetimes, but for the moment I want to empha-size a very simple fact that obsessive past-life selves often forget, namely: that past life is done! As I often say in workshops to people who get caught up too strongly in the thoughts and passions of their past lives, the best reason to remember most past lives is to forget them. Or to put it even more simply, in the words of Jalaludin Rumi: A Sufi knows that the past is completely over!

Despite the pain and struggle and karmic imprints of so many difficult lives, our memory banks also hold vivid stories of peaceful lives in which we died painlessly in our beds, surrounded by loving companions—"a consummation devoutly to be wished" (Hamlet again). People with past-life experiences of this kind report gently floating into higher realms in the afterglow of a well-lived life, to be greeted by loving beings of light, often ancestors. The Tibetan tradition counsels us that the finest way to die is leave this transient world consciously and peacefully if we can, taking no thoughts, no feelings, no body pains of any kind with us; it teaches us that only when we become completely empty can we know the pure radiance of our limitless minds.

When you do the next CD exercise, either type of life may come to you: a life of struggle or a life of peace. Both have their learnings; both have their opportunities for healing. In these wise verses, William Blake summed up the deep reconciliation we can reach with the peaks and valleys of our earthly life:

Man was made for joy and woe;
And when this we rightly know,
Thro' the world we safely go.
Joy and woe are woven fine,
A clothing for the soul divine.

CD TRACK 3
Exploring a Past Life and Going beyond the Death
This exercise will take you more directly into a past life and give you an opportunity to see the outline, if not all the details, of a complete lifetime. You will also be guided to experience the ending of that lifetime, and to go through and beyond the death experience. There is nothing to be afraid of in the exercise itself. However vivid the death, what you see, hear, and feel will only be images in your memory. Your body and your surroundings will remind you all the time

where, in fact, you are today. But be prepared for some strong feelings, as you would if you were watching a very engrossing movie: maybe fear, maybe deep sadness, possibly physical reactions. These are all part of the old story. Your ego self will be present throughout the exercise as a witness; you can always say to yourself, if the images and reactions you have are very strong, "This is only a memory," just as you can say during a powerful movie, "These are only actors on a set!"

In the next chapter and in the next exercise on the CD (Track 4), you will be able to continue work with any "unfinished business" from the particular past lifetime you encounter here.

As in the previous exercises, prepare yourself with headphones if you like, a notebook, and drawing materials. Now find a quiet place where you will not be disturbed, and listen to Track 3 on the enclosed CD.

CHAPTER
FIVE

Between Lives:
Healing in the Bardo

id he live his life again in every detail of desire, temptation, and surrender during that supreme moment of complete knowledge? He cried in a whisper at some image, at some vision—he cried out twice, a cry that was no more than a breath, "The horror! The horror!"
                                                                    —Joseph Conrad, *Heart of Darkness*

... nd over there, beyond the grave, we shall say that we've suffered, and that we've wept, that we've had a bitter life, and God will take pity on us. And then ... we shall begin to know a life that is bright and beautiful, and lovely. We shall rejoice and look back on these troubles of ours with tender feelings, with a smile—and we shall have rest!
                                                                    —Anton Chekhov, *Uncle Vanya*

REVIEWING A PAST LIFE: THREE BASIC QUESTIONS

In the last chapter, I gave several examples of how it is possible in your past-life regression to pass over to the spirit realm, or bardo state, after death. By now you have probably been able to envision the essential events of a complete past life, including your own memory of the death transition that followed it. You have probably begun to glimpse that extraordinary state of consciousness that the soul experiences when it reaches the other side. You may have seen yourself dying peacefully, or violently, or prematurely, but in each case, you have had the sense of leaving the dead body and going to another place, another state of awareness.

If you have not already done so, either spontaneously or deliberately, it is very useful to review the past lifetime, particularly the circumstances and state of mind in which you died. As I emphasized in Chapter 4, the state of mind of the dying person produces the strongest karmic patterns to be passed on to subsequent lives. By taking time to consciously and carefully review themes and issues that you died with in that life, you can not only understand the essence of your soul's unfinished business, or karma, from that other life, you can also take steps to clear it.

The most effective way to clear your karmic patterns from a past-life regression is to ask yourself, or have a past-life therapist ask you, three basic questions:

1. What am I thinking at the moment of death?
2. What am I feeling at the moment of death?
3. Do I have strong physical sensation or pain at the moment of death?

These simple but pointed questions will help you focus on all the major imprinting you took with you from that life. They address three levels of human experience that correspond to three different vibrational levels of the subtle body: the mental, the emotional, and the physical. (In Chapter 6 we will explore the imprints of subtle-body memories in more detail.)

These questions are also the first step to clearing the state of confusion that the departing soul frequently finds itself in immediately after death. Sogyal Rinpoche explains this state as the typically accelerated activity of the mental body, which obsessively re-runs the events preceding death—but after the death, it does this on the other side, in the bardo, not realizing that the life is really over. Such states of confusion can be cleared at death by certain funeral rites, urging the soul to let go and to move on, but if the confusion was not cleared in the past life, that part of the soul still clings to its memories of life and all of its unfinished business. This aspect, this fragmented part of the soul stays stuck in its angry, terrorized, or confused condition, fixated, we would say in Freudian terms, in this state of mental and emotional obsession. The patterns belonging to this un-integrated fragment are re-imprinted and re-run over and over in other lives, long after their original context is forgotten.

LAST THOUGHTS AND FEELINGS IN THE BARDO STATE

The mind is its own place, and in itself
Can make a Heav'n of Hell, a Hell of Heav'n. ——John Milton, *Paradise Lost*

When someone is killed violently or dies prematurely, he or she will inevitably have many conflicting and unresolved thoughts and feelings at the time of death; only a Gandhi or a Christ can face death with complete compassion and equanimity. Whether or not there is physical trauma at death, there is usually powerful emotion: deep grief at the loss of children or loved ones, rage at the injustice of betrayal or exile, and often vows of terrible vengeance. We may die ashamed and humiliated following some punishment or banishment. In a lifetime as a failed leader, we may feel so agonizingly responsible for the suffering and death of others that we die consumed with guilt. Our minds react with great passion and with great anguish: we cannot let go of our moments of horror, agony, or despair, and we cling to the memories of these painful scenes, inexorably creating new karma and binding ourselves ever more tightly to the wheel of rebirth.

Such thoughts and feelings, if they are present with great intensity when we die, will follow us with undiminished intensity into the after-death realm of the first bardo. Hindu and Buddhist wisdom has always known this sad but fundamental fact of transition. Emmanuel Swedenborg, the great Swedish visionary whom D.T. Suzuki called "the Buddha of the West," rediscovered it in the eighteenth century and wrote in his *Heaven and Hell*:

After death a person is engaged in every sense, memory, thought and affection he was engaged in in the world: he leaves nothing behind except his earthly body.

So it is no surprise that much of the confusion that souls find themselves facing in the bardo is generated primarily by their feeling states and negative thoughts, which can be so powerful that they blind the transiting soul to its new state of being. Many feel caught in the endless reiteration of rage at their persecutors; others seem lost in a cloud of despair or depression; still others seem determined to hide, tormented by overwhelming guilty thoughts such as "I could have prevented their pain."

HEDDA: RELEASING WRITER'S BLOCK
A Greek Philosopher Whose Books Were Burned

Hedda's story offers a striking example of how limiting a thought left over from a past life can be. Hedda wanted desperately to write novels. She was very talented, but she had severe writer's block and could not get any of her novels finished. Instead, she would be overcome with inexplicable lassitude and a despair that undermined all of her creativity. When Hedda went to a past life, she found herself as a different kind of writer, a philosopher in ancient Greece, at a time when the Romans were invading. The philosopher had spent all his life accumulating and copying and creating philosophical texts, and he had collected a remarkable library—until the Romans came, attacked his village, and burned the house down with all the manuscripts inside. The writer died distraught, all his works of philosophy gone. He was so depressed, so angry and unhappy, that he said, toward the end of that life, "I'll never write again."

In the regression, Hedda became very strongly aware of this thought in her—"I'll never write again"—and saw that it belonged not to her, but to the past-life personality who lived within her, the personality of the ancient Greek philosopher. She had to talk to him, bargain with him a little bit, and say, "The Romans aren't coming today. It's okay to write again; it's safe." When she did this, she found she was able to get on with her writing, and in a way, to get on with *his* writing, because it was unfinished business, with some philosophical insights that still needed to emerge.

I have witnessed more than a thousand regressions, and I have come to the conclusion that the departed soul in distress needs very much the same kind of therapy it lacked on the earth: a chance to vent feelings, to release grief or shame, to ask for forgiveness, or simply to find some spiritual reconnection with that which was lost. The bardo becomes a place where we have the opportunity to heal through simple spiritual psychodramas that allow the cathartic release of feelings, the possibility of reconciliation with enemies we had conflict with on Earth, or reunion with those we have been separated from.

WENDY: BEYOND THE MASSACRE
A Spiritual Homecoming

When we met Wendy in Chapter I, we saw how the Native American boy's tragic story of failing to save his family had a devastating impact on her life today, leaving her with lifelong panic attacks when she was separated from her own family. Her story illustrates how complex the feeling states and negative thoughts carried over into the bardo can be. At the same time, it also shows how they can be resolved through simple psychodrama, reflection, and what the old spiritual traditions called metanoia, which is to say, a change of heart.

In Wendy's story, you may remember, the young boy and his father returned home just in time to see the mother and younger children killed by soldiers. Despite a heroic attack, the father and son were themselves slaughtered. During the regression, I asked the key questions to bring the imprinted patterns to light: "What are you thinking and feeling as you die?" The boy's dying emotions were a terrible mixture of anguish and grief, fear and guilt; his overriding thought was, "I should never have left them alone."

For a while, in the bardo, Wendy discharged huge amounts of grief as she replayed the images of the boy's mother, brother, and sister lying on the ground. Her body still trembled with the young boy's terror when he himself was seized and killed. She sobbed uncontrollably. "I should never have left them! How could I do that?"

"Where are you now?" I asked her.

"I'm still there, looking at the bodies," she sobbed. "I just can't believe it!"

I asked how long she stayed there. "Many days," she said, "but now the vultures have almost finished with them. It's horrible."

"What happens?"

"I'm leaving now. I'm floating above, high above the village. But I can't stop thinking about what we did, how foolish we were."

"Are you alone?" I asked.

"I don't notice anyone else. All I can think about is how we let them die. It's all our fault."

"It's all over now," I tried to reassure her. "Be aware of that."

"I'm never going to forget," she said. "That must never happen again."

To break Wendy out of the negative self-absorption of the boy's guilt, I told her, "You're not in a body now. Nor are they. Look around you? Who do you see?"

She broke into tears again as the boy spoke: "It's my father. He's reaching out to me. He's telling me not to worry. There was nothing we could have done. We were totally outnumbered. It's hard to hear him, but then he beckons me. 'Look,' he says, 'they're all here!' And they are! My mother and the little ones. They are all shining and beautiful; their faces are radiant. They seem to know it's over better than I do. 'You're never going to lose us,' they're saying. My goodness!

I recognize them: it's my three children from this life!" At once she saw, on a deeper level than ever, what her anxiety had always been about and why she felt so bereft when the children left home, one by one.

In this moving psychodrama, I gave Wendy a cushion to hold, and she asked for more cushions as she hugged all the spirits of the lost family. Caught between laughter and tears, she exclaimed, "They're telling me I'm not to blame, I'm not to blame! The whole village is there. They're having a big dance around the fire. It's like they're welcoming me home." And so they were!

RELEASING FEELINGS: THE POWER OF CATHARSIS

Most of the time, in our more dramatic past-life death scenarios, our feelings are indistinguishably fused with our thoughts as we die. As you begin to recognize your own past-life stories, you may start to see how strong feelings attached to situations in your current life, such as hatred, resentment, self-doubt, jealousy, or suspicion, have their origin in past lives. The second basic question—"What was I feeling at the moment of death in that lifetime?"—helps us realize how many of our persistent feeling complexes are actually projected from a "story behind the story." Ask yourself:

- Am I still angry with the people who brutalized my family?
- Am I still in despair that I was separated from my loved ones?
- Do I feel unhappy that the life somehow was a failure?
- Am I still brooding over something I deeply regretted?
- Are my feelings of being shamed still holding me back from being fully in life?

As you review your past lives, become aware of those feelings that you are still carrying. You will need to tell yourself that the life where they arose is finished.

Those emotions are no longer appropriate; they are no more than emotional residues it is time to let go of, if you can. You may need to express these feelings to release them fully. Perhaps there is some crying to do. Perhaps there is some raging. Perhaps you need to forgive yourself for something that you did and regretted. You have an opportunity now to reflect on the past and take away its emotional charge.

MAXINE: PROFESSIONAL KARMA

A Journalist Driven by Past-Life Injustice

When I met Maxine, it was not hard to see how she was driven by anger. She cared passionately about all the injustices she saw around her. Living in South America and working as an investigative journalist, she was never short of work, and spent much of her time rooting out political scandal and secret diplomacy stories. In her past life, she found herself as a Mexican revolutionary in one of the wars at the end of the nineteenth century. This revolutionary had been captured by the Spaniards and executed without a trial, tied to a post and shot.

As we replayed the story in a psychodrama, the revolutionary in Maxine relived the rebellious death, angrily straining at the ropes that held his wrists, blindfolded and full of anger and hate. The dying thought was, "I'll never let this happen again." Indeed, that is what Maxine was attempting to do today in her work as a journalist. It was not necessarily a bad carryover, professionally speaking, but she did need to release a lot of the anger held in her wrists and jaw, which did not all belong to the political scandals of today. Confronting the Spanish tyrants in the bardo gave the revolutionary in Maxine a lot of satisfaction, as well as the insight that there was still karma to be completed.

JUAN: FEAR OF A FATAL MISTAKE

The Boy Who Was Hanged for Stealing Bread

Juan, a social worker, consulted me because he suffered from severe performance anxiety: he hated to speak out in public. The greatest challenge for him was to give reports about his social work cases in front of a group of colleagues. He was always terrified of them ridiculing him, criticizing him behind his back. He was convinced that he would make some terrible mistake in front of them—although nothing remotely like this had ever happened.

We started Juan's regression using the most loaded phrase for him: "I'm going to make a mistake. I'll get it wrong." As he lay on the mat, his emphasis quickly changed: "I've made a mistake," he said. "I've done something wrong. I'm going to die!" His whole body went rigid and his hands spontaneously went behind his back.

"What's happening?" I asked. "Where are you?"

"They're all looking at me. It's awful. I'm so ashamed. I've done something they tell me is wrong."

"What did you do?"

"I've stolen," he said. "It was bread. I was starving. And now I'm going to die."

Juan found himself in a medieval European town as a ten-year-old boy who had been caught stealing and dragged before a magistrate. Condemned to hang, he was marched through the street as a crowd of townspeople jeered at him. He hung his head in shame. As he mounted the scaffold, his body got more and more tense. In a miniature psychodrama, I gently suggested the hangman's rope with a folded towel around Juan's neck (using absolutely no pressure). Suddenly, he convulsed, his back arching. He choked, went quite blue for a moment, and fell back on the mat, limp.

Then the tears came—and the rage! "How could they do that? I never hurt anyone. There was never any work. No one gave a damn about us on the street.

I hate them! I hate them!"

"See them all," I instructed him.

"I see that pompous, hypocritical judge! You disgusting, heartless pig! And the burghers—so fat and comfortable in their furs and finery. What did they ever care about us poor?"

I let Juan rage for a while, knowing that this sense of injustice was at the root of all the fear and all the humiliation. Then I asked, "Are they all like that?"

"No, not at all. Many of the townspeople know me and like me. They're telling me it was nothing! It's just the rich protecting their interests. They don't blame me. Life isn't fair! The rich rob and steal with impunity.

"The ordinary people are all gathering round me now in the spirit world," he went on. "I feel good with them. They actually admire me, how I survived for so long on the streets; I see that I was orphaned. No wonder I chose social work as a profession today! They're telling me I must speak out against social ills, that I should be proud of my work. I feel much stronger now. Phew, to think I was carrying all that." He felt his neck. "This has always been stiff," he said, "and I hate turtleneck sweaters and ties!"

I tightened the towel around his neck a little. "Pull it off," I said. He did so, firmly. "Now your neck is free," I told him.

Juan called me some time later to say that all of his anxiety at public presentations had gone—and guess what? He had been asked to give talks at a local youth facility, and he had actually enjoyed it!

In both of these past-life stories, the bardo, or after-death, was essentially a place to let go of old emotional, mental, and physical patterns. Simple forms of psychodrama helped Maxine and Juan to express their grief, their rage, and their pain, encouraging them both to go beyond their fear to a place where they knew with great clarity and reassurance that the past was truly over. Much more than that, by connecting with the spirits of those they had known on earth, they broke old patterns and began to forge strong new behaviors that pulled them out of the compulsive repetition of old suffering.

CD TRACK 4
Clearing Memories of Past-Life Deaths and
Finding Reconciliation in the Bardo

In the previous exercise you encountered—and went beyond—your death in a past life. You are probably comfortable now with being above or beyond the past-life death scene. You have started to develop the "heavenly eye" and to work in the bardo state.

But there may be many things that still feel unfinished from the past life you have explored. This exercise will help you clear these issues by suggesting a wide range of questions to ask yourself, elaborating on the three basic questions about unfinished thoughts, feelings, and physical sensations. You will also be helped to contact guides and spiritual teachers to gain even deeper insights into your experience.

As before, prepare yourself with headphones if you like, as well as a notebook, pen, and drawing materials for recording your journey and the messages you receive. Now find a quiet place where you will not be disturbed, and listen to Track 4 on the enclosed CD.

CHAPTER SIX

How Our Bodies
Remember Past Lives

We entered the house of realization,
We witnessed the body.
—Yunus Emre

The body keeps the score
—Bessel A. van der Kolk

SUBTLE BODY MEMORIES: THE ETHERIC IMPRINT

When we go deeply into a regression, we often have extraordinarily vivid memories of physical pain, contortion, struggle, or disempowerment, and we experience all this in a fully embodied consciousness. To feel the phantom pain of having a sword in the side, or of being raped or beheaded, puts us in touch with the deepest level of traumatic residue that has persisted across lifetimes. In the previous chapter, Juan vividly relived a hanging death, which had lain frozen in the stiff neck he had suffered from all his life. Elmore's chronic back pain held the memory of a savage beating (Chapter 3); Madeline's guilt from her life as a slave master imprinted a similarly morbid memory in her neck and shoulders (Chapter 4).

Such physical memories often shock us when they surface in a regression, especially when there is nothing to account for them in the current life. The most helpful explanation is that these memories are embedded in the subtle body—literally, the layers of subtle energy that surround and penetrate the physical body. (Some researchers have called it "cellular memory," but this metaphor unfortunately raises more questions than it answers. The Russian research into the bioelectrical auras around plants, animals, and human bodies, which can be recorded with the technique of Kirlian photography, is more descriptive, speaking of "energy fields" in and around the body, like magnetic fields.) Both past-life research and past-life therapy have now collected an impressive array of evidence to show that these old traumas, inherited though the first level of the subtle body—which I will also call the *etheric field* or *blueprint*—consistently re-imprint in the living body as rashes, deformities, birthmarks, weaknesses in certain limbs, or organic disorders such as a weak bladder, a weak heart, gynecological problems, and so on.

WOUNDS FROM THE PAST

The devastating effect of past-life physical wounds imprinted on the subtle body at the etheric level cannot be overestimated. It is in many ways the most radical discovery to be made in past-life regression work, and it has the potential to revolutionize the way we approach physical healing. Here are some examples of how healing does, in fact, take place when the past-life wound is remembered and released in the etheric field:

• Sophie had suffered from migraine headaches for many years. During a workshop, she recovered a past life as a young girl in a nineteenth-century mining town out west. Her father, an alcoholic, frequently molested her and brutalized her. On one occasion, she answered him back, and he took an iron bar and hit her over the head, crushing her skull. When Sophie relived this horrible death, she felt a brief "splitting headache" as the bar cracked open her skull. Then she was beyond the body, looking down at it and at her now remorseful father. As her spirit moved away from the dreadful scene, she felt a huge lifting of energy from around her head. From that day on, her migraines never recurred.

- Pedro suffered from chronically stiff shoulders and a very tight back that no amount of chiropractic or bodywork ever seemed to relieve. In a regression to a prehistoric past life as a South American peasant, he found himself captive to an ancient priestly tribe that was using most of his tribe for slave labor to build temples and pyramids. He suffered many years of hardship, carrying heavy basket-loads of rocks up the slopes. He was forever under the eyes of overseers, who viciously lashed any slaves who stumbled or slowed in their work. One day his body gave out and he collapsed, partly paralyzed, with compacted spinal vertebrae, never to work again. Left to starve, he died bitterly, in terrible back and shoulder pain. But once his spirit reached the bardo, he could look down and see his body and know that he no longer had to do that literally backbreaking work. After a healing psychodrama in which he simulated pushing a heavy weight off his back, Pedro reported that his shoulders and back felt totally different. The pains did not return.

- Flavio suffered from chronic arthritic pain in his hips and right leg. Although much of the pain was around the joints, he also reported that his right leg was always tense from the knee to the hip. Rather than try to detach him from his pain, as many therapies do, I took the approach of allowing the painful leg to produce a story by exaggerating the tension. Flavio quickly saw himself as a navy man in the eighteenth century whose ship was being bombarded. His lower right leg had been shattered by a cannonball, and the ship's surgeon was amputating it above the knee. Two strong sailors held him down as he screamed in agony. This was the tension causing the terrible pain in his right leg and hips: he was trying with all his might to pull his leg away from the surgeon's saw.

He died not long after from massive blood loss and trauma, but his body struggled to the very last. When Flavio saw himself above the ship and the sea battle, he was by no means out of the story; his body still trembled with the phantom pain.

In the workshop psychodrama, I had three strong men role-play the surgeon and his helpers. The tension immediately redoubled as they held Flavio down.

"They're taking my leg!" he screamed.

I asked him, "What is your body trying to do?"

"I'm trying to hold onto my leg!"

I let him pull and pull to experience the extent of his fight to hold on. Then I instructed the role-players to let go, so that Flavio could pull his leg away from them. In doing this, he collapsed, exhausted. All the tension was gone. "Look," I said. "You haven't lost your leg today; it's still here!" But he had needed to complete that huge unfinished battle to save his leg: an old struggle that had been locked in his leg and hip muscles by the etheric imprint of that awful death.

Healing of physical/etheric trauma takes place in the bardo through detaching from the old scene—knowing that it is over, deciding to let go—and using a variety of spiritual or imaginary strategies to reorganize the subtle body itself. In Pedro's and Flavio's cases, a psychodrama of having the load removed or the leg reclaimed was enough to transform the frozen residue of pain for both of them; it erased the old program, the old tape that had been running in their unconscious minds and bodies.

RECOGNIZING AND CLEARING ETHERIC WOUNDS

To capture the last moments of physical struggle before dying, distressing as it often is, is paramount in the healing process. The third key question I suggested for reviewing your past-life regression experiences is extremely helpful in recognizing these physical/etheric patterns: "Do I have strong physical sensations or pain at the moment of death?"

When you reviewed a memory of dying in a previous lifetime (Track 4 on your CD), you were invited to see yourself leaving the body of the past-life personality and encouraged to ask yourself: "Am I still carrying anything in this remembered body? Am I still feeling any pain from that death or from an earlier physical experience in that lifetime, possibly abuse, possibly abandonment, possibly starvation?" If you find that you are, try to talk very gently to that part of your body. Say simply, "It's over. You can let go of the pain now." The pain embedded in your energy field may not "know" at its own level of consciousness that the experience is finished. The self-protective pattern (rigid back and shoulders) or the pattern of terror (tense stomach, producing ulcers) is still being replayed in the body as a somatic blockage, tension, or illness. But you can tell that part of your soul's memory, "It's all over. You're no longer a slave being abused. You're no longer a tribal villager being run through with a Conquistador's sword." Whoever that character is, we need to tell him or her that it is time to let go of the story and its imprints at all levels, in the mental, emotional, and physical energy fields where they are held.

There is a second type of psychodrama that can be useful for healing deep etheric wounding. Many people who die severely wounded in a past-life death find themselves conducted by spirit helpers in the bardo realm to a sort of spiritual hospital, where they receive various forms of healing, often entailing light. Sometimes a spirit animal will come to suck out poison, clean a wound, or strengthen an area of the subtle body with some of its own energy. (Healing of this kind is well known among traditional shamans, many of whom talk of working with the luminous body; the knowledge that healing can take place in the subtle, or luminous, body is axiomatic to them.) Similarly, in regression healing in the bardo, we can often help replace severed heads, severed limbs, or burnt skin, or close gaping wounds using transfusions of light administered by spirit healers and spirit animals. The spiritual imagination has tremendous power to heal in these higher realms, or bardos, which vibrate at a higher frequency than the material world.

ROSANNA'S SPIRIT HEALING

Rosanna suffered from various gynecological problems and a difficult history of childbearing; each of her pregnancies had been fraught with complications that led to Caesarian deliveries. While she loved having children, being pregnant had been a series of nightmares for her every time. She wanted another child, and so did her husband, but not with so much pain around the process. When she did some past-life sessions, she saw herself in more than one life dying in childbirth—scenarios that, in themselves, left her with a lot of fear—but the worst memory was of a pregnant woman whose child was taken from her for a ritual sacrifice. So cruel was this society that they cut the child out of her before she came to term. This was the deepest and most painful imprint she was carrying, and it was clearly associated with her repeated Caesarians.

In the regressions, at first Rosanna went out-of-body at the death scene, which was all too understandable, but when she finally relived the death in the body, she felt how deeply she had held tension and terror in her abdomen all her life, and how it underlay her problems in that part of her body today. When she went to the spirit world, a loving group of ancestors—the Grandmothers, I will call them—came to meet her. Her lost baby was there, and she was tearfully reunited with him. Then the Grandmothers took her to a sacred waterfall, where they healed her subtle body by sewing up her mutilated belly and cleansing her pelvic and genital wounds. All the while, they gently sang to her their ancient tribal songs.

THE FOUR SUBTLE ENERGY FIELDS

When we envision the subtle body as a number of different energy fields, it helps us see with greater precision the different kinds of "unfinished business" that can imprint during a difficult past-life death and surface in a past-life regression. To help you as you go on with your own regression work, it may be useful to review the fields, or bodies, I have referred to most often, outline the issues typically associated with them, and show again how they interact to form a powerful imprint of a past life.

Drawing on the traditional yoga teachings of the ancient Indian sage Patanjali, we can distinguish:

- **The etheric or vital field** This carries the imprints of all physical wounds, injuries, mutilations, sicknesses, or body pains not healed or resolved in a particular lifetime. This field is quite close to the physical body, and carries all the meridians known to Chinese acupuncture and similar systems. Its chief energy form is *qi* or *prana* or simply *life force*. When it is blocked or carrying scars from the past, the living energy cannot flow, and illness or dysfunction arises.
- **The emotional field (or astral body)** This carries vivid memories of all unresolved feeling states and emotional traumas from past lives, such as fear of physical violence, anger at injustice, depression about a hopeless situation, grief at deep loss, guilt at cruel behavior, shame from abuse or humiliation, or worthlessness from having failed in some way. This field

extends two or three feet around the physical body and can be sensed or clairvoyantly "seen" as a person's *aura*, often in colors corresponding to feeling states or moods.

- **The mental field (or mental body)** This carries all obsessive and repetitive thoughts, such as "I'll get back at them," "No one cares about me," "I should have done more," or "There will never be enough." It also carries thoughts that have a negative or limiting impact on the self, thoughts that often directly perpetuate states in the emotional body: "I'm no good, I failed them," "They're all watching me," or "I'll never trust anyone again." This field is many feet around the body, sometimes filling a room or even an auditorium.

We are already familiar with these three fields because they correspond to the emphasis of the three basic questions regarding thoughts, feelings, and physical sensations at death. But there is a fourth field that transcends the lower three:

- **The spiritual field (or causal body)** This subtle field does not, strictly speaking, belong to the individual, but relates to what Jung called the *collective unconscious* beyond individual consciousness; through it, outside spirit forces influence or penetrate the other subtle bodies. In this field, we find any remnants of psychic and spiritual connections, positive or negative, to the spirits of people we were strongly involved with in a particular past lifetime. These are the karmic ties that bind us to others, and they can have profound repercussions for our current life when we recognize them. The spiritual field may hold energies that interact with any or all of the other bodies in various ways. For example, spirits of dead children from a past life may attach to the uterine area of the etheric field; spirits of lonely or unhappy beings we once knew may attach to grieving parts of the emotional field; wronged or abandoned spirits may angrily attach to the mental field, which still feels guilty about betraying them.

The first three levels of energy, the mental, emotional, and vital or etheric bodies, lift off as a total energy envelope at death. They are a bit like Russian dolls, where you get a grandmother doll and open her up and there is a smaller mother inside, and then you open her up and there is yet a smaller one, and finally you get to a little baby in the middle. So imagine that the physical body is like the baby. The first level to peel off in the death process is the outer layer, the mental body. This is the energy field that carries, so Patanjali says, the imprinted, embedded thoughts. Then comes the emotional body, which carries the imprinted feelings. The final level to lift off, the level closest to the physical body—the smallest doll enclosing the baby in the Russian doll model—is what we call the *etheric body*, the vital or life-energy body.

So when a person dies, these three levels of imprinting go with him or her. If someone has been stabbed in the back, the etheric body, the smallest of the bodies, will carry with it an imprint of that stabbing, which becomes an etheric blueprint, influencing future lives at the physical level. Even an image of the knife will stay embedded in the subtle body at the etheric level. Now if the person who was stabbed was very angry at the time—if, for example, he was killed in a fight in a bar—there will be a deep imprinting of anger in the emotional body connected deeply to that wound in the etheric body. (The anger might be seen clairvoyantly as red energy around the spot where the person was stabbed.) This angry energy is further out in the field than the physical/etheric imprint of the stab wound, but the imprints are connected by images of the event. There may be other residues in the emotional field as well, not necessarily connected with the death trauma. For example, if the person lived a very lonely life, alone in his village with no friends, there may be bitterness in the emotional field attached to images of loneliness.

The third level of imprinting that lifts off at death carries the thoughts—the whole mental universe—of the dying individual. (Doubtless this accounts for the myth that the whole life of a drowning man flashes before him.) The man who dies in the barroom brawl with a knife in his back is thinking angrily, "I'll get back at him. I'll kill him. How dare he do this to me?" These thoughts are emotionally charged, but they are thoughts nevertheless. They are specific ideas of revenge held, so Patanjali would say, in the outer sheath of the energy body, the mental body. When such vengeful thoughts belong to the mental imprint, they drive the emotional field and embed themselves in the etheric blueprint that is carried to subsequent lives.

The fourth level of energy, the spiritual body, cannot be said to "lift off," because it is outside the individual, belonging to the collective unconscious rather than to an individual consciousness, but its influence is felt after death in memories of unfinished business, remnants of relationships, and connections with the psyches of others who have died. (A general who dies consumed with guilt over the deaths he has caused may be haunted by memories and even by the spirits of those fallen soldiers in the spiritual field.)

All these energies, imprinted in the aura of a future body, contain frozen or compacted images of the life in which they occurred. Regression work, as well as energy transmission, meditation, and many types of bodywork and healing, can bring fragments of these images, usually charged with feeling, to the surface. And when we understand the ways in which the energy of a past life—mental, emotional, physical, spiritual—imprints in the different fields of the subtle body, we can regress and review with even more nuanced attention, adding a fourth question to the basic three:

"What am I thinking at the moment of death?"
"What am I feeling at the moment of death?"
"Do I have strong physical sensation or pain at the moment of death?"
"Who am I unfinished with at the moment of death?"

I end with an example that shows clearly the different levels of subtle-body imprinting and how each influences the others in the residue of a past life.

CARMELLA: A HEART MURMUR
Unending Loyalty to a Great Leader

Carmella, a young journalist, was very conscientious at her job, yet she was a rather lonely person, still searching for the right man in her life. She was quite anxious about the physical dimension of past-life work when she saw it demonstrated in a workshop, and she asked me if it was safe, since she was taking medication for a mild heart murmur. I told her not to worry, and she underwent a regression that did indeed focus on her heart pain. She found herself as a soldier loyal to a Scottish pretender to the English throne in the early seventeenth century. The pretender invaded England, but the campaign failed, and the loyal soldier was left for dead with a pike through his chest, close to the heart. He died in agony, thinking in his delirium, "I mustn't leave my beloved lord; I must stay with him. I mustn't leave my post." As the soldier left his body, his spirit did not go into the spirit realm at all, but hovered around the body it had just left, repeating, "I mustn't leave my lord." In this state of confusion, the spirit of the loyal soldier really did not know that he was dead.

First, I reminded the soldier's spirit that he was, in fact, dead. Then I asked Carmella the three basic questions: "What pain are you still carrying from that lifetime in your body?" "What are you feeling?" "What are you thinking?" She identified the pike in the soldier's heart, and I suggested she imagine a spirit helper to pull it out. Now Carmella started to weep, and it was clear that the huge physical pain in the heart region was compounded by the emotional wretchedness the soldier felt at losing his beloved master. And at the mental level, thoughts that "I have to be with my lord" were keeping his spirit locked in an imaginal repetition of the dying moments on the battlefield. He was unable to move on because—as he repeated obsessively—"I mustn't leave my post." Eventually, I persuaded him to go and find his lord in the spirit world, and to be acknowledged by him. In doing so, he was able to answer the fourth question, "Who are you unfinished with?" and heal the karmic wound of that severed connection in the spiritual field. There was rejoicing as he found himself once more in the service of his beloved master—whom Carmella recognized as a mentor in her own life today.

After unburdening so much sadness, Carmella felt greatly freed in her heart region. Some months later, she called to tell me she had stopped taking medication for her heart murmur altogether. She even wrote up her story in a local magazine.

CHAPTER
SEVEN

Making Our
Souls Whole

Countless lives inhabit us.
I don't know, when I think or feel,
Who it is that thinks or feels.
I am merely the place
Where things are thought or felt.
I have more than just one soul.
There are more I's than I myself.

—Fernando Pessoa

 man to be greatly good, must imagine intensely and comprehensively;
he must put himself in the place of another and of many others;
the pains and pleasures of his species must become his own.

—Percy Bysshe Shelley

THE MANY MASKS OF THE SOUL

The more we work with our past lives, the more we come to see that we carry within ourselves a whole cast of characters—a set of selves that one Jungian writer, Jolande Jacobi, has called the "masks of the soul." To become fully human is to recognize, and even to experience, extremes of our nature that can range from sublime heroic heights to the depths of depravity.

To grow morally and spiritually, we must see that we have in us both the hero and the villain, the seductress as well as the saint; that both creator and destroyer, tyrant and exile are part of our soul's repertoire. We must learn to see our own shadow. As Carl Jung put it, "We do not become enlightened by imagining beings of light, but by making the darkness conscious."

When our past-life explorations bring to light a difficult past life, a shadow life, we may want to reject or suppress it, especially if it does not sit comfortably with the more favorable image we have of ourselves. But if we can find a way to live with this unpleasant "other," there eventually arises within us a kind of creative tension between the opposing selves. "Without contraries is no progression," wrote William Blake, and the same is true in the soul: painful as this tension may be, it sets in motion a spiritual dynamic through which the soul can grow into its higher potential for love and compassion.

Now that you have begun to record and review your own past-life stories, you may notice how the theme of one life often reverses itself in another life in a play of psychological opposites. You might recall a past life as a peasant in a village ravaged by brutal warlords, then in the next life find yourself a ruthless Conquistador invading, raping, and pillaging. It is as though your soul has role-reversed from powerless victim to powerful aggressor.

From all of the cases of regression I and my coworkers have recorded, it is clear that the twin poles of any archetypal complex—in this case, power—do, indeed, reverse themselves in this way, swinging across lifetimes like a pendulum from one extreme to the other. This dynamic of action and reaction is, of course, what Eastern teachings call *karma*. In remembering our past lives, we experience firsthand how the karma we carry today was originally laid down and transmitted through various lives. We might see, for instance, how our difficulty making money today arises from a life where we squandered a lot of money and died guiltily blaming ourselves, saying, "I never should have had all that money! It didn't make me happy."

FROM PROCONSUL TO PEASANT

Scepter and crown
Must tumble down
And in the dust be equal made
With the poor crooked scythe and spade.

—James Shirley

Guy was a typical example of how, in regression work, extreme polarities that are in conflict within the soul manifest in life after life, compensating (or overcompensating) for each other. Though he had a pronounced tendency to arrogance in his present life, Guy never rose very high in the ranks of the corporation where he worked for many years. He seemed unaccountably held back, despite grandiose—though not impractical—visions of how he would run the firm if it ever fell to him.

Then, in a major regression session, Guy had a memory of being Proconsul of Spain in Roman times—pretty much the dictator of Spain on behalf of the Roman Empire. He had power over the whole of that territory, and was answerable only to the emperor. There was a sense of grandeur and vastness in this life of Guy's. He was a big man physically, and he had enormous power, with thousands of subordinates, legions of soldiers, and a whole political structure beneath him. But in the next life he recalled, he found himself as a peasant in medieval Holland, living in a tiny shack on a tiny plot of land, barely twenty feet by twenty. He spent that whole life in his little village, scratching out a living in the most wretched of circumstances, with a few chickens and a pig. He had gone from one extreme of power and control over vast territories to the opposite extreme of restriction and limitation. Guy's soul needed to experience those opposites as part of a long lesson in humility.

Other stories from my case files show the same dynamic at work:

- Ramona remembered the painful past-life experience of being raped by soldiers on a battlefield. She was powerless and humiliated, and she died extremely angry. Her dying thought was, "I'll never let this happen to me again. I want to kill them." In the next lifetime she flashed upon, she saw herself dressed in rough clothes and leather and metal armor. She was a warrior, in fact a Viking, invading villages in the north of Europe, killing and raping. She had reversed from the victim to the perpetrator, and she was making sure it never happened again—to the Viking, at least. Recognizing this progression helped Ramona see how angry she was at men in her present life and how heavily defended—armored—she was in her body.

- Dagoberto saw himself as a Jewish victim of the Inquisition, deeply humiliated, then tortured to death as a heretic. Then he saw himself returning in a subsequent lifetime to be a powerful judge in a small German town, where he had the power to condemn people to death, torture, and other cruel punishments. In this progression, he saw the source of the deep compassion he feels today for all victims of persecution, but he also recognized a judgmental side in his present personality—for example, toward Arab suicide bombing of the Jews in Israel.

- Helga, who had undergone open-heart surgery not long previously in this life, saw herself in a past life as a priest in a South American culture. The priest's job was to sacrifice children, and it was done by cutting out their hearts. The inescapable connection with her own surgery led to a catharsis. Helga realized that she had been unconsciously carrying enormous guilt from the priest's life, and that despite all the selfless work she had been doing with very sick and dying children as a nurse in a children's hospital, she had never been able to lay it to rest. She had actually brought on her heart condition by overwork, precipitating what turned into a felicitous healing crisis.

EXPLORING THE POLARITIES OF YOUR SOUL

The opposite is what is good for you.   —Heraclitus

The next exercise on the CD gives you an opportunity to explore some of the past-life polarities in your own deeper soul history. You will start with one of the lives you have already accessed, then be guided to look at a life that represents its opposite. So, if you have already seen a painful life, I will encourage you to experience a more pleasant one. But if you have already seen a simple, quiet life, the exercise will challenge you to look at a more complex life, possibly a difficult one. This work with opposites bears out Jung's idea that the opposite self, the shadow self, needs to come to light. It is not always easy to look at a shadow life—a life where we have done harsh things, a life where we feel unworthy or guilty—but if you can do so, it will be profoundly healing. It is like finding a piece of you that has been hiding in the darkness, waiting, if you are willing, to be redeemed.

CD TRACK 5

Balancing Past Lives

In this exercise, you will be guided to recall one of the exercises you have already done, one in which you found your way deeply into a past life or in which you got an overview of a story, understanding most of the events of that life and where they led you. You will be encouraged to remember how you died in that life, and to remember, too, how you passed over to the other side, into the bardo realm.

You will recall how, possibly, you needed to talk to the spirits of people you had known in that life, to finish things that were incomplete, to express certain thoughts or feelings, to heal certain wounds in your subtle body. Then you will be helped briefly to review the life and its chief theme from the bardo perspective. Finally, you will be given suggestions for moving into a very different kind of life—an opposite life—to see how your soul reversed that theme.

As you have done in all of the previous exercises, prepare yourself with headphones if you like, a notebook and pen, and drawing materials for recording your journey and any messages you receive. Now find a quiet place where you will not be disturbed, just as you would for meditation, and listen to Track 5 on the enclosed CD.

INTEGRATING AND HEALING YOUR PAST-LIFE SELVES

In the deserts of the heart
Let the healing fountain start.   —W.H. Auden

When we start to integrate a pair of opposing life stories, either by reviewing them in the bardo or by reflecting on them over time, we begin a major spiritual work. By bringing to consciousness that part of the soul that lay unfinished in your previous life or death, we infuse it with fresh energy, so we can embrace life with a newer and wiser perspective. A wounded part of the soul is healed; a lost, prodigal part is found. As our practice of past-life remembering progresses, we may discover different levels of understanding at different stages of the journey. The work can extend over many years, becoming what Jung called the *opus magnum*, the true alchemical transformation of the soul.

On an energetic level, if we can get deeply in touch with emotions and sensations that arise when we remember our past lives, we can also bring the emotional and physical energies within the subtle body back into balance. By working consciously on scars from past-life wounds, and by unfreezing memories locked in fearful places in our present bodies, we can promote the release of strong "streams" of energy in our subtle bodies. Chronic areas of stiffness may dissolve as we let go of physical and emotional burdens we have been carrying from past lives, no longer relevant to our current life. Blocked libido may begin to flow naturally again as we let go of old bitterness and resentment that has been blocking our ability to give ourselves freely and passionately to another—the result of betrayal or abuse in a previous life.

On a psychological level, equally important healing takes place when we recognize the patterns of self-blame, self-limitation, vengeance, shame, or self-criticism we have been harboring from our past-life stories. We come to see these patterns as bitter but deeply human reactions from painful past lives—lives where we did appalling things, made shameful decisions, or wretchedly failed our fellow beings. When we face these stories honestly and openly, seeing them in the human context in which they arose, then we can entertain them compassionately and let them go. We recognize that our past lives are precisely that: past. And we find that we have it in us not only to forgive others, but ultimately to forgive our (other) selves.

As the Tibetan masters have always known, the process of conscious dying offers us the supreme opportunity to let go of the negative karmic patterns buried deepest in our souls. Whatever we can let go of as we cross the threshold of death into the bardo is left behind, not passed on. And in just the same way, when we rework memories of dying in previous lives, we have a second chance to erase that psychic residue from the karmic slate. Sogyal Rinpoche teaches that birth and death are one cyclical process, all part of the endless transformations of Universal Mind. Once we understand this—and once we remember our soul's past "intensely and comprehensively," in Shelley's words—we can start to let the ever-flowing river of being wash away the negative accretions of our lower, self-ridden nature. Through this process of purification, our energy fields become lighter, less dense, as we shed the karmic residues and psychic debris we have carried for lifetimes.

The great teachers tell us, too, that if we can relinquish our attachment to the whole business of personality—in this life and across many lives—our ego will eventually be stripped of all its paralyzing obsessions and delusions. Such a practice of "self-naughting," the mystics say, marks the beginning of the soul's ultimate journey to know the Divine. Then we come to see that all these characters, all these stories that we carry from our past lives, are nothing more than the masks of the soul, cast away when the drama ends. When we see this, we are ready to do as Rumi says:

Renounce all the faces in your heart,
So that the face without a face may come to you.

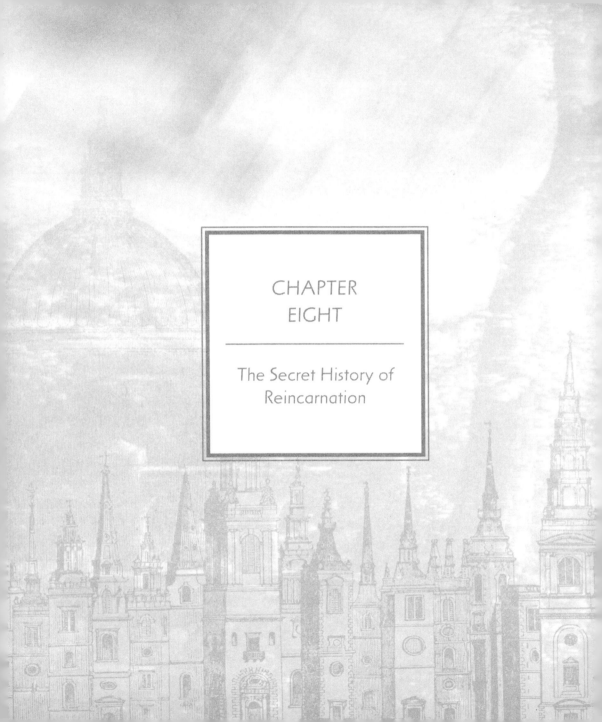

CHAPTER EIGHT

The Secret History of Reincarnation

Worn-out garments
Are shed by the body:
Worn-out bodies
Are shed by the dweller
Within the body.
New bodies are donned
By the dweller, like garments.
—Bhagavad-Gita II

NOT LONG AGO, I saw a slogan on a bumper sticker: "Reincarnation is having a comeback." It is a sad fact that the scientific establishment in the United States still marginalizes most work that even hints at realities beyond our own, including regression therapy, parapsychology, and a vast body of research into paranormal phenomena, from out-of-body experiences to children's spontaneous past-life memories. By clinging to such a narrow protocol, mainstream psychology risks becoming, in George Orwell's memorable phrase, one of "the smelly little orthodoxies which are now contending for our souls." Fortunately, in most countries where I have lectured, the general public is far ahead of the academics. Nearly everyone has heard of the doctrine of reincarnation, and recent polls show that almost one in three Americans now believes in it, even though most of the Christian churches reject it.

In recent years, a number of influences have brought past lives into present consciousness. The widely read writings of Edgar Cayce, for example, have been surprisingly influential in America, lending credence to the idea that past lives can contribute to illness, emotional difficulties, relationship difficulties, and so on. (I say "surprisingly" because Cayce channeled thousands of past-life readings while in a trance state, even though his fundamentalist Christian conscious self did not initially believe in past lives!) Many people, thanks to Cayce, now understand the idea of karma as the spiritual fallout of good or bad behavior from the soul's past. Still others have encountered Hindu teachings, in which the idea of reincarnation is central, by being exposed to yoga or by reading the popular works of authors such as Caroline Myss and Barbara Brennan on the chakras, the subtle bodies, and energy medicine. The famous Hindu text *The Bhagavad-Gita* is for sale today in nearly every bookstore.

And who would have expected to see the Dalai Lama vying with the Pope in the bestseller lists? The high-profile presence of Tibetan Buddhist lamas throughout America and the world has profoundly altered the spiritual landscape of Western society. The making of a film like *Little Buddha*, with its story of a Tibetan lama reborn in the body of a young American boy, would have been unthinkable in Hollywood a generation ago, but now it receives huge acclaim. Nor does an actor like Richard Gere hesitate to profess his Buddhist affiliations publicly. Many people, myself included, have turned to meditation and radically changed our lifestyles after exposure to these powerful emissaries of ancient wisdom.

WHO BELIEVES IN REINCARNATION?

A better question might be, "Who doesn't?" The influx of traditional teachers and teachings from the East clearly accounts in part for our shifting attitudes toward reincarnation, but over the centuries the West has had many distinguished believers of its own. Take the following delightful example:

The body of B. Franklin,
Printer,
Like the Cover of an Old Book,
Its Contents Torn Out
And
Stripped of its Lettering and Gilding,
Lies Here,
Food for Worms
But the Work shall not be Lost,
For it Will as He Believed
Appear Once More
In a New and more Elegant Edition
Revised and Corrected
By the Author

Benjamin Franklin's witty epitaph for himself, written supposedly when he was twenty-one, was never used on his tombstone, but it remains one of the most succinct and memorable summaries of the idea of reincarnation ever penned. Franklin did not have his tongue in his cheek, either. At eighty-eight, he wrote to a friend, "I look upon death to be as necessary to the constitution as sleep. We shall rise refreshed in the morning."

Nor was Franklin the only famous Westerner to believe that the soul not only survives death but returns in a new body to continue or to rectify the life previously lived on earth. Evidence of this belief can be found in the writings of poets, writers, and philosophers across centuries: Dante Alighieri, Marsilio Ficino, Paracelsus, William Shakespeare, Johann Wolfgang von Goethe, William Wordsworth, Emanuel Swedenborg, David

Hume, Arthur Schopenhauer, George Sand, Walter Scott, Victor Hugo, Ralph Waldo Emerson, Richard Wagner, Walt Whitman, Emily Dickinson, W.B. Yeats, Aldous Huxley, Somerset Maugham, D.H. Lawrence, Rainer Maria Rilke, Pearl S. Buck, Carl Jung, Winston Churchill, Norman Mailer, and Shirley MacLaine.

REINCARNATION, CHRISTIANITY, AND PAGANISM

Reincarnation has never officially been condoned by the Catholic Church or any of the major Protestant churches, but it was an almost universal belief among the many Gnostic and pagan sects that proliferated in the first three centuries of our era. Most educated Greeks and Romans of the Hellenic period subscribed to it, especially those initiated into the great Mystery schools of Eleusis, Mithras, Dionysus, or Osiris. We find it in the teachings of the Pythagorean brotherhood, an offshoot of the Orphic mysteries, and, of course, in the doctrines Plato taught in his famous Academy. The philosopher and initiate Plutarch, who became a priest at Delphi, wrote, "We know that the soul is indestructible and should think of its experience as like that of a bird in a cage. If it has been kept in a body for a long time and become tamed to this life as a result of all sorts of involvements and long habituation, it will alight back to a body again after birth and will never stop becoming entangled in the passions and chances of this world."

Many surviving Gnostic writings, whose origins are hotly debated by scholars, show striking similarities to Buddhist and Hindu teachings about the soul's journey after death, no doubt because of many centuries of contact between Eastern and Western cultures following the conquests of Alexander the Great. (It is known, for example, that Buddhists taught in Alexandria and that yogis reached Athens, where they were dubbed the gymnophysicists.)

Before the third century C.E., pagan and early Christian beliefs existed side by side in the Roman Empire, but when the emperor Constantine adopted Christianity as the religion of the state, the Gnostics and the Mystery schools came in for persecution, and reincarnation came to be seen as a heresy. Reincarnation was finally excised from Roman Church thinking in 553, when the teachings of Origen about the preexistence of the soul were anathematized by the emperor Justinian. After this, it disappeared from Church history for nearly one thousand years, briefly entering Europe as part of the teachings of the Cathars, the late Gnostic group that flourished in Northern Italy and Southern France in the twelfth and thirteenth centuries. Considered a threat to orthodoxy, the Cathars were brutally extirpated by the Church in the notorious Albigensian Crusade, which spawned the Inquisition (and in which my past-life mercenary plays a small but ignominious part).

SECRET TEACHINGS AND INITIATES

In the East reincarnation survives, buried within Hermetic and Platonic teachings that are secretly preserved by certain monastic orders during the rise of the Orthodox Church in Byzantium. These teachings, along with hundreds of lost manuscripts, came west again in the fifteenth century, when Cosimo de Medici acquired the collection for his famous Academy in Florence, modeled on Plato's own. This priceless library of ancient texts—among them, famously, the lost books of Plato—laid the intellectual and spiritual foundations of the Renaissance.

But the fearful years of the sixteenth and seventeenth centuries, the Wars of Religion in Europe, forced many of the Hermetic teachings underground once more. They were carefully disguised in the opaque symbolism of alchemy and in Rosicrucian allegories that only initiates could penetrate;

one such initiate, who surely knew of reincarnation and a great deal more, was William Shakespeare. (Others were the painters Albrecht Durer, Sandro Botticelli, and Leonardo da Vinci, the poet Edward Spenser, and the English magus Dr. John Dee.)

From the Renaissance on, with the rise of rationalism and early science, the psyche of the West began to split. More and more, rationalist philosophers attacked anything spiritual as superstition. In the eighteenth century, John Locke proclaimed that the mind is a *tabula rasa*, a blank slate, at birth. Building on this dogma, as we saw in Chapter I, the burgeoning "science" of psychology would eventually decide to throw out any idea of psychic inheritance, or inborn memories or traits, thus breaking with three thousand years of wisdom gleaned from the ancient philosophy of the soul. (Perhaps it is no coincidence that this doctrine appeared just as all of Europe and its land-grabbing settlers were trying to disown flagrant acts of colonial aggression, genocide, and the horrors of slavery. With events like these to remember, collective memory could prove embarrassing!)

THE HERITAGE OF THE ROMANTICS

But side by side with the growth of scientific rationalism, whose achievements within its own domain should never be underestimated, we see the appearance of the great Enlightenment explorers of the soul—Emanuel Swedenborg, Franz Anton Mesmer, Johann Wolfgang von Goethe, Friedrich Wilhelm Joseph von Schelling—followed by the "visionary company" of the Romantic movement, as Harold Bloom has called them: William Blake, Samuel Taylor Coleridge, Percy Bysshe Shelley, John Keats, and William Wordsworth. A generation after Locke's tabula rasa, Wordsworth penned one of the great affirmations of the soul's "eternal return":

Our birth is but a sleep and a forgetting;
The soul that rises with us, our life's star,
Hath had elsewhere its setting,
And cometh from afar;
Not in entire forgetfulness,
And not in utter nakedness,
But trailing clouds of glory do we come
From God, who is our home.

In fact, it is this "alternative" (actually, Neoplatonic) philosophy of the soul, declared by the Romantic poets all over Europe and later taken up by the Transcendentalists in New England, that lays the groundwork for the study of the deeper soul that nineteenth-century philosophers began to call the *unconscious*. And this whole rich tradition, fired by Freiderich Nietzsche's dismantling of the Christian psyche and Arthur Schopenhauer's sense of a divine Will (imported from the Hindu *Upanishads*), leads us straight to Sigmund Freud, Carl Jung, and the psychoanalytic movement: the closest thing the modern world has seen to an authentic science of the soul.

THE PERENNIAL QUESTIONS

Where do we come from? What are we? Where are we going?   —Paul Gauguin

At various points in its increasingly conservative history, mainstream psychology, with a zeal worthy of the early Church casting out heretics, has thrown out the soul, thrown out spiritual and psychic experiences, and even come close to throwing out the personal testimony of subjective experience—all with that deadly Behaviorist movement that is still stifling research today.

To this day, Freudian psychoanalysis is heretical at most universities; Jung is taught only at more radical institutions. Yet we do not have to look far to see that the idea of the unconscious mind as the repository of the soul's experience is still very much alive. Thanks to Thomas Moore's bestseller *Care of the Soul*, inspired in part by his great mentor James Hillman, we can now talk more openly about the soul. And thanks to transpersonal psychology, with its appreciation of "altered states of consciousness" (Charles Tart), the manifest benefits of meditation; the "spectrum of consciousness" behind our spiritual evolution (Ken Wilber), the soul's memories before birth (Stanislav Grof), the psychic journeys of the shaman (Michael Harner), and the healing power of imagery (Joan Borysenko), we can seriously boast a growing science that is neither narrow nor dogmatic.

These are the traditions from which I write and which have influenced my thinking and my practices for several decades. With Jung and the transpersonalists, I believe that only by studying the religious dimension of the psyche can we fully appreciate the greatest mysteries of our being. And once we truly acknowledge the primordial reality of the soul, which by far transcends our limited human personalities, I believe we can address the questions that have always challenged humanity: "Where do we come from?" "What are we?" "Where are we going?"

BOOKS

Bowman, Carol. *Children's Past Lives: How Past Life Memories Affect Your Child.* New York: Bantam, 1997.

A fine account of what children have to tell us. Contains many provocative stories and summarizes the work of Dr. Ian Stevenson.

Hall, Judy. *Thorsons Principles of Past Life Therapy.* New York and London: Thorsons, 1996.

An excellent short account of past-life regression as a therapeutic tool.

Head, Joseph, and S.L. Cranson. *Reincarnation: The Phoenix Fire Mystery.* New York: Warner, 1979.

An encyclopedic book that is indispensable for anyone researching reincarnation in world history.

*Lucas, Winafred Blake. *Regression Therapy: A Handbook for Professionals.* Two volumes. California: Deep Forest Press, 1993.

Remains the state-of-the-art compendium of both the theory and the techniques of regression therapy for any therapist or healer.

Sogyal Rinpoche. *The Tibetan Book of Living and Dying.* New York and London: HarperCollins, 1992.

This beautifully written book (co-authored by Andrew Harvey) is by far the most accessible work on the bardo teachings of Tibetan Buddhism by a practicing living master.

*Woolger, Roger J. *Other Lives, Other Selves.* New York: Bantam, 1987.

Essential reading for a deeper understanding of the entire regression process. Considered by many the authoritative work on past-life regression therapy.

AUDIO

Woolger, Roger J. *Jungian Past-Life Therapy.* Boulder, Colorado: Sounds True, 1992.

Recorded at a public seminar in London, this audiotape includes a live demonstration of a past-life regression by Dr. Woolger.

Woolger, Roger J. *Eternal Return: How to Remember and Heal Your Past Lives.* Boulder, Colorado: Sounds True, 1992.

A greatly expanded version of much of the material in this book. This audiotape includes a powerful live session of a complete regression session.

VIDEO

*Woolger, Roger J. *Other Lives, Other Selves.* Connecticut: Hartley Film Foundation, 1994. (U.S. version only.)

Excerpts from a workshop for therapists, illustrating the remarkable power of past-life regression. Contains dramatic examples of the regression process.

RELATED WRITINGS BY DR. WOOLGER

(Downloadable at www.rogerwoolger.com)

"Body Psychotherapy and Regression: The Body Remembers Past Lives." In *Body Psychotherapy,* edited by Tree Staunton. London: Brunner-Routledge, 2002.

"Deep Memory Process and the Healing of Trauma" with Andy Tomlinson. Woolger International, 2003.

"The Presence of Other Worlds in Psychotherapy and Healing." In *Thinking Beyond the Brain,* edited by David Lorimer. Edinburgh: Floris Books, 2002.

WORKSHOPS, PROFESSIONAL TRAINING, AND SESSIONS WITH DR. WOOLGER

Roger J. Woolger offers public workshops and professional training in the United States, Europe, and Brazil in Deep Memory Process, his form of regression therapy. Please visit his Web site at www.rogerwoolger.com.

Information about workshops, training, and TK sessions may be obtained from the following offices:

Woolger International (U.S.)

51 Elting Avenue, New Paltz, New York 12561

Phone: 845-255-0515, Fax: 845-255-0517, Email: woolgertraining@aol.com

Woolger Training (U.K.)

Briarwood, Long Wittenham OX14 4QW

Phone and fax: 01865-407996, Email: woolger.uk@talk21.com

*These titles may be ordered directly from www.rogerwoolger.com.

Roger Woolger, Ph.D., is a Jungian analyst, past-life therapist, and professional lecturer with degrees in psychology, religion, and philosophy from Oxford University and London University. He trained as an analyst at the C.G. Jung Institute, Zurich. Dr. Woolger has served as a visiting professor at Vassar College, the University of Vermont, and Concordia University in Montreal. He is the author of *Other Lives, Other Selves* and co-author, with Jennifer Barker, of *The Goddess Within.*

SOUNDS TRUE was founded in 1985 with a clear vision: to disseminate spiritual wisdom. Located in Boulder, Colorado, Sounds True publishes teaching programs that are designed to educate, uplift, and inspire. With more than 500 titles available, we work with many of the leading spiritual teachers, thinkers, healers, and visionary artists of our time.

For more information on Roger Woolger, or for a free catalog of wisdom teachings for the inner life, visit www.soundstrue.com, call toll-free 800-333-9185, or write: The Sounds True Catalog, PO Box 8010, Boulder CO 80306.

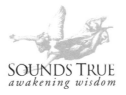

SOUNDS TRUE
awakening wisdom

CD SESSIONS

1. A Memory Exercise:
Re-Imagining Childhood Games 9:00

2. Exploring Personal Difficulties:
An Emotional Release Exercise 13:00

3. Exploring a Past Life and Going Beyond
the Death 9:00

4. Clearing Memories of Past-Life Deaths and
Finding Reconciliation in the Bardo 26:00

5. Balancing Past Lives 18:00